Metaphor and Meaning in Psychotherapy

Metaphor and Meaning in Psychotherapy

ELLEN Y. SIEGELMAN

THE GUILFORD PRESS
New York   London

Printed in the United States of America

This book is printed on acid-free paper.

Last digit is print number: 9 8 7 6 5 4 3 2

Library of Congress Cataloging-in-Publication Data

Siegelman, Ellen.
    Metaphor and meaning in psychotherapy / Ellen Y. Siegelman.
      p. cm.
    Includes bibliographical references.
    ISBN 0-89862-431-2   0-89862-014-7 (pbk.)
    1. Metaphors—Therapeutic use. 2. Symbolism (Psychology)
3. Psychotherapy. I. Title.
    [DNLM: 1. Psychoanalytic Interpretation. 2. Psychotherapy—
methods. WM 420 S571m]
    RC489.M47S54 1990
    616.89'14—dc20
    DNLM / DLC
    for Library of Congress   90-2726
                                  CIP

For Mitzi and
for Charles,
enhancers

Acknowledgments

The seeds of this book were planted many years ago by my parents' interest in the written word and by a series of gifted teachers in high school, college, and graduate school. Perhaps the most outstanding and formative of these was the distinguished American man of letters, Robert Penn Warren, from whom I was fortunate enough to take courses in creative writing and in the analysis of poetry. His attention to the technical resources of poetry—rhyme, meter, tone, diction, and above all, imagery and figurative language—catalyzed my lifelong passion for the products of the imagination.

After obtaining my doctorate in psychology, I took postdoctoral training in the Psychiatry Department of Mt. Zion Hospital, an interdisciplinary training program that drew on the faculty of the San Francisco Psychoanalytic Institute to give its trainees an unusually rich and diverse understanding of the practice of psychoanalysis and of psychoanalytic therapy. Many years later, feeling the need to go beyond this training in a different way, I was accepted by the C. G. Jung Institute of San Francisco for their analytic training program, allowing me to explore systematically the other great depth psychology of our day.

To the faculty and staff of all these programs, and particularly to my personal and control analysts, I want to express my gratitude.

I am indebted to the Psychotherapy Institute of the East Bay for inviting me to be an annual symposium speaker in 1984; my talk at that symposium became the nucleus for this book, and it was expanded in a course I taught for therapists at that institute on working with dreams and metaphors in psychotherapy.

More specifically, in the writing of this book I have had the benefit of support and close readings from a number of friends and colleagues. Hilde Burton, Emily Loeb, Naomi Lowinsky, and Peter Siegelman generously read the manuscript in its entirety and offered especially thoughtful comments. A number of others commented usefully on parts of the book, including Sue Elkind, Stephen Joseph, Peter Rutter, Stephen Siegelman, and Philip Siegelman. Mitzi McClosky has been the book's presiding angel from the very beginning, offering her special brand of confidence and encouragement that helped me over the rough places.

Sandra Wooten, a gifted bodywork therapist, has deepened my firsthand experience of the connection between the body and symbolic experience.

Finally, I want to thank my patients. They have not only given me the rare privilege of sharing their deepest lives but have corrected me when I was wrong and have left with me a treasury of metaphoric images. I have drawn on their material abundantly in this book, trying to preserve its thematic sense and flavor while being careful to preserve their anonymity by extensively compositing and by disguising all identifying details. I know that case examples can be used manipulatively (Samuels, 1989); I have used them not to prove but to amplify and to suggest.

Permission to use quotations from lines of verse or extended quotations from prose works has been generously granted for the following publications: *Forms of Feeling*, Robert Hobson, copyright 1985 by Robert Hobson, reprinted by permission of Tavistock Publications; *Luisa Domic*, George Dennison, copyright 1985 by George Dennison, reprinted by permission of Harper & Row, Publishers, Inc; "As I Walked Out One Evening," W. H. Auden, from *The Collected Poems of W. H. Auden*, copyright 1976 by Edward Mendelson, William Meredith & Monroe K. Spears, reprinted by permission of Random House, Inc. "Little Gidding," by T. S. Eliot, from *Four Quartets*, copyright 1943 by T. S. Eliot (renewed 1971 by Esme Valerie), reprinted by permission of Harcourt Brace Jovanovich, Inc.

A portion of Chapter 8 was first published, in somewhat different form, in *The Journal of Analytical Psychology*, Vol. 35, No. 2 (April, 1990) and is reproduced by permission of the Society of Analytical Psychology, London

Preface

Metaphor making—the imaginative act of comparing dissimilar things on the basis of some underlying principle that unites them—is one of the ways we construct a new reality. By its very nature, metaphor combines what is already known in a new way to produce a new thing not yet fully understood. In this book, I propose to give an anatomy of metaphor as used by therapist and patient in depth psychotherapy.

My two decades of experience with patients have shown me that salient metaphors, or those that can be made salient through exploration, have three important characteristics:

1. They often—Arlow (1969b) would say *always*—represent "the outcropping of an unconscious fantasy."
2. They combine the abstract and the concrete in a special way, enabling us to go from the known and the sensed to the unknown and the symbolic.
3. They achieve this combination in a way that typically arises from and produces strong feeling that leads to integrating (i.e., affectively grounded) insight.

I will attempt in this book to document with case examples the truth of these assertions. In examining both the nature and the power of metaphor, I will show how its clinical usefulness can be maximized. As we shall see, even seemingly dead or inert metaphors can, like Lazarus, be brought back to their life-giving source.

In addition to heightening consciousness about understanding and using metaphor in clinical work, I want to show that the entire encounter of a depth-oriented psychotherapy can be understood metaphorically and that that understanding enriches our work. For what distinguishes depth therapy from other kinds of psychological treatment (supportive, behavioral modification, counseling, suggestion) is the symbolic attitude that informs its conduct. This is true of the ritualized context in which it operates as well as the therapeutic relationship. Indeed, the central metaphor in depth therapy is the transference.

I came to psychology with a passion for the literary imagination and with advanced training in literature. Although poets and patients are very different in the skill and deliberateness with which they use metaphors, the underlying imaginal processes are similar. Moreover, many depth therapists have a poet's feel for the heightened emotionality of figurative language. This book is an attempt to set down in a fairly systematic way what many of us do intuitively or unthinkingly. In becoming more conscious of how we and our patients use metaphors, we can more effectively understand and deploy them.

I bring to this book not only a literary perspective but years of research in personality and child development, and clinical training and experience in the major depth psychologies. In my own work, I have tried to honor the best of Freud and Jung and object relations theory (particularly the British middle school). Within the Jungian fold, I am closest to those Jungians who emphasize early development along with that "something more" that is the symbolic in its richest sense. As will be apparent, I am against reductionism of any kind, because, satisfying as any "nothing-but" explanation may be, it does violence to the complexity of inner life.

In citing Jungians with increasing frequency in the course of the book, I hope to provide a bridge that helps further the interchange between the various schools of depth psychology.

Indeed, if one central metaphor has shaped the book, it is the image of the bridge. Metaphor is essentially a bridging operation, and bridges do not reduce, they connect. Jung (1931b) called symbols (the larger class to which metaphor belongs) "bridges thrust out towards an unseen shore." The unseen shore can be thought of as the unconscious as well as the unseen. Metaphors offer a passageway to the unconscious, not perhaps the royal road of dreams, but an important thoroughfare, nevertheless. They also serve as bridges between affect and insight, since the hallmark of a living metaphor is the intense feeling that surrounds it. Metaphor is a way to mobilize and release affect. Because it uses the concrete and visual, which is the first language any of us know, it has powerful connections with the unconscious. And because all metaphors are connecting operations (connecting one term with another), the work of the conscious ego is involved as well. Metaphor is thus an ideal vehicle for embodying both conscious and unconscious, both affect and cognition.

An interest in bridges (bridges between Jungians and Freudians, bridges between conscious and unconscious) leads not only to the land masses that are connected but to what is in between. This in-between, third thing is what Jung (1916) talked about in the acts of imagination that mediate between conscious and unconscious and what Winnicott (1971) later designated as the transitional space, which is midway between fantasy and reality and is the domain from which art and culture spring.

A part of my larger purpose is to join my voice to those who have reacted against a too narrow or disparaging view of primary process among classical Freudians. We view these acts of reverie and figurative expression not as default operations or sublimations but as deeply satisfying intrinsic characteristics of what it means to be human.

The shape of this book also is quite consciously like that of a suspension bridge. The first two, somewhat more theoretical chapters are like pylons supporting the central span. They ground the book in theory, define terms, and set out some of the larger issues surrounding metaphor. Chapters 3 through 7 are like the central span of the bridge: clinical chapters that draw heavily on actual metaphors as used effectively and ineffectively by patients and by therapists. The last two chapters lead to the other shore—the world of the symbolic of which metaphor is a part: the domain of fantasy, of play, and of creativity.

Plan of the Book

Chapter 1, "The Primacy of Metaphor," establishes the "pedigree" of metaphor, showing how primary and ubiquitous it is in thought and in language. An attempt to salvage "primary process" from the disparagement it has suffered shows how works of the imagination are not just regressions or sublimations but useful mediating enterprises. A section on the importance of affect in metaphor concludes the chapter, which includes examples from cases and from fiction.

Chapter 2, "The Bodily Matrix of Metaphor," also addresses the primacy of metaphor by exploring the body—the source of our sense experience—as the ground of many of our metaphors. This leads to a discussion of psychosomatic symptoms and their symbolic meaning and of the differences between symptom and metaphor. It concludes with a case example of how a psychosomatic symptom came to be understand and thereby converted into a metaphor.

Chapter 3, "Exploring Clinically the Unconscious Sources of Metaphors," uses examples of moment-by-moment process within the therapeutic hour to show how metaphors that seem automatic, conventional, or casual can be resuscitated if listened to with a discerning third ear. It suggests how a seemingly unimportant figure of speech, when welcomed and allowed to expand, can reveal itself to be a statement of a patient's general psychological situation. It further demonstrates the importance of a patient's first-time use of a novel metaphor.

Chapter 4, "Metaphors of the Self: Changes in the Course of Therapy," again draws on clinical examples to show how the therapeutic changes that took place in two patients reflected and were further shaped by the key images they used to describe their lives. Changes in such overarching self-metaphors can be used as markers of the success or stalemate of the therapeutic process.

Chapter 5, "Metaphor and Defense," concerns itself first with the metaphors used defensively by patient and therapist when there is some need to speak in a metaphoric "code." It also deals with the metaphors by which patients reveal their defensive systems. Particular attention is given to spatially constricting metaphors (of which the prison is the prime example) and to images of spatial openness or diffusion. These are shown to be analogs of psychological states.

Chapter 6, "The Therapist's Metaphors," turns to interpretations or heuristic statements cast in metaphoric terms; considers the question of when a therapist shares his or her own internal image; and looks at the ideal case, with an example in which patient and therapist jointly weave a metaphoric construction. The importance of a therapist's image as a valuable countertransference cue is also exemplified in this chapter, as is a brief discussion of the metaphoric base of empathy.

Chapter 7, "Pitfalls in the Use of Metaphor," discusses two kinds of clinical pitfalls—both the overvaluation and the underappreciation of figures of speech, each of which has unfortunate consequences for therapy. It also addresses a broader metaphoric pitfall that applies to our theoretical templates: the tendency to freeze or literalize metapsychological metaphors and take them as the truth rather than as working hypotheses or constructions.

Chapters 8 and 9 are the final pylons that support the clinical bridge on the far end.

Chapter 8, "Metaphors of the Therapeutic Encounter," considers the large-scale metaphors used by Freud, Jung, Langs, Milner, and Winnicott to describe the therapeutic interaction and the therapeutic space. The consequences or "entailments" of these metaphors for the therapeutic process is suggested, as is the different flavor that practitioners of different styles attach to the same figure (e.g., "the frame").

Chapter 9, "The Symbolic Attitude," anchors the bridge in the larger domain of meaning. A description of the symbolic attitude so necessary to the depth psychologist leads to a consideration of failures in the symbolic attitude in patients. That failure is described as an inability to play, and attention is given to how to foster that capacity. An exploration of the similarities of the symbolic attitude and the aesthetic attitude leads to the formulation of a musical metaphor for the psychotherapeutic process. The book concludes with a final case example in which music and affect are movingly linked.

I would hope that by traversing the bridge of this book, the reader will become increasingly aware of the riches waiting on the unseen shore.

Contents

CHAPTER 1

The Primacy of Metaphor

Metaphor is a tool so ordinary that we use it unconsciously and automatically, with so little effort that we hardly notice it. It is omnipresent: metaphor suffuses our thoughts, no matter what we are thinking about. It is accessible to everyone: as children, we automatically, as a matter of course, acquire a mastery of metaphor. . . . And it is irreplaceable: metaphor allows us to understand ourselves and our world in ways that no other modes of thought can.

GEORGE LAKOFF AND MARK TURNER, More Than Cool Reason.

"Life's . . . a tale told by an idiot." "My cup runneth over." "I'm drowning in my tears." "My past is full of ghosts."

Metaphors such as these—drawn from poets and from patients—exert enormous power over us. And the capacity to express one thing in terms of another is not just the property of poets, though they use these figures more deliberately and more skillfully than others do. Most of us, and our patients as well, in moments of strong, inexpressible feeling, find ourselves cleaving to metaphor to communicate experience that is hard to convey in any other way.

Let me start with the metaphor of a patient:

CASE EXAMPLE

He sits in the chair opposite mine—a middle-aged man who sighs frequently and whose sparse hair is rumpled. He is telling me about his father's family, the Rosenthals (I have disguised the actual name). They were great practical jokers, he says—lively and funny. And they had no patience with anyone who was soft or shy, obviously referring to himself. "Toughness—that was the watchword in Rosenthal-land."

Rosenthal-land. He was creating a metaphor in front of me: A family is a country. The idea excited me. A family *is* a country, I thought to myself: Each family has its own mores, its own tribal customs, its jingoism and xenophobia. Did his have passports and entry visas? Did it declare war on other family countries? But most of all, I wondered, what rules bound the citizens of this country?

"And what were the laws of Rosenthal-land?" I asked.

He cocked his head, perhaps surprised that his submerged metaphor was being taken literally. The wordplay appealed to him, and being a lawyer and fluent with words, he proceeded to rattle off the laws of the family country:

"Well, let's see. There was: 'Nice guys finish last.' And there was 'Never give a sucker an even break.' And 'If you give someone a finger, they'll take a whole hand.' And, hmmmm, there was, 'Do them before they do you.' And most of all, there was the law that said, 'Big boys don't cry.'

"Goddamn," he went on, hitting his fist on the chair. 'It sounds awful."

"It sounds like Sicily under the mafiosi, that country," I said.

"Yeah. I guess I never saw that quite so clearly till now. What a lousy country for a kid to grow up in!" He rubbed his forehead, and thought for a while, and when he began talking again, the feeling atmosphere in the room had changed.

He was remembering his mother's funeral when he was 13, how he had wanted to stay with the coffin and keep them from putting on the last of the dirt, and how he had begun to cry. "You've got to be tougher than that," his father had said, pulling him away from the grave. And that memory, which grew out of the metaphor, brought tears to his eyes. He wept in sorrow and frustration and longing.

A family is a country: The therapist who brings a heightened consciousness and involvement in and with the metaphor will find that it unleashes buried affect, buried insight, and a way of making the past present and the unconscious conscious. This book is an exploration of how that happens.

WHAT IS "PRIMARY"?

Webster defines "primary" as "first in order of time or development, or in intention; primitive, original; fundamental" and as "first in dignity or importance: chief, principal." It is in both these senses that metaphor is primary. I will try to show that metaphor is primary both in language and in thought. It is through metaphor that we come to understand the world and through metaphor that language itself develops. Furthermore, the capacity for metaphor making is linked with the primary process in psychological development and has its origins in the way young children apprehend the world.

Metaphor is "primary" not only in the chronological sense but in its importance as well. As the quintessential "bridging operation," metaphor links domains by connecting insight and feeling, and what is known with what is only guessed at.

The metaphorical shape of this chapter is, I hope, a web in which the central node is "primacy." The filaments radiating out from it will connect with language and child development, the symbol-making bent of our psyches in sleep and wakefulness, and how our patients communicate what is primary to them. Along the way, I will outline the anatomy of metaphor and compare the dream image and the metaphoric image.

METAPHOR AND THE ORIGIN
OF LANGUAGE

According to Lakoff, (1987), Lakoff and Johnson (1980), and Lakoff and Turner (1989), we are not simply given our world but we "construct" it through our perception and categories of thought. Metaphor is basic to such construction. I am increasingly drawn to their idea that metaphor is not just a figure of speech but an elementary structure of thought. They have identified a series of basic metaphors (e.g., life is a journey, death is a destination, time is a changer) that we require to think about the most basic human experiences. These metaphors draw on what we have experienced concretely in journeys, destinations, and changes, and "map" those experiences onto their respective abstract "target domains." Such generic metaphors eventually become so automatic and conventional that we use them without realizing they are metaphors at all. The kinds of comparison I will be using in this book are generally of a more image-laden, less conventionalized sort, but they are, nonetheless, important in structuring how we understand our experience.

Being basic to thought, metaphor is also basic to the language we use, since language embodies our conceptual understanding. Language expands primarily by comparing the known to the unknown, so we can probably assume that language is essentially metaphoric. In *Philosophy in a New Key*, a book that is as important now as when it was published in 1948, Susanne Langer studied the symbolism of reason, ritual, and art. She held that the main way in which we develop new ideas is through the metaphoric process. Essentially, that process entails describing one thing in terms of another so that from this comparison a "third thing," the new idea, is born. This is as true of similes ("A is like B") as of the more dramatic metaphor ("A is B").

Indeed, it seems that we can *only* see the new at first in terms of the old: Something completely and totally new would be not only indescribable but incomprehensible. And it is a basic property of the mind to seek to attach new perceptions to old contexts, to seek analogies. How often when meeting a new person do you think, "He reminds me a little of so-and-so?" or "This street corner in Paris reminds me of the corner with that little church at 12th Street and Fifth Avenue New York"? Langer goes so far as to say that "every new experience, or new idea about things, evokes first of all some metaphorical expression."

As a metaphor becomes familiar, it becomes conventional and automatic. If we say, for instance, "I was seething with anger," we may not picture our body as containing hot liquid about to boil over. Nevertheless, this metaphor has been mapped into a basic one based on our bodily experience: Anger is heat in a container. When you are angry, your heart pumps, you feel hot and flushed, your "gorge rises." What Lakoff (1987) has called a "source domain" (the realm of our bodily experience) has been "mapped into" a more abstract "target domain" (the emotion of anger); in this way, we increase our ability to comprehend and communicate about the feeling.

Or we can think of certain image-metaphors that have become conventional. "Head" is applied to tables as well as people. A cap as a headcovering becomes metaphorically generalized to any similar covering such as a hubcap or to "capping" an oil well. Although such metaphors have become conventional and some writers have referred to them as "dead" or "faded," Lakoff and his co-authors believe that they are in fact more essential and alive when doing their work in our language unconsciously and automatically. As I will show in Chapter 3, metaphors that are used conventionally and without awareness by our patients can be explicitly reconnected, through exploration, to their vital sources in sensation and feeling.

The Anatomy of Metaphor

Langer (1948) characterizes metaphor as "our most striking evidence of *abstractive seeing*, of the power of human minds to use presentational symbols" (p. 114). It uses concrete sensory experience (primarily visual) to convey an abstract idea. When Marc Antony in *Antony and Cleopatra* decries the desertion of the friends who once had "spaniel'd me at heels," we see through the image-metaphor of the dog the kind of devoted—even fawning—attachment he is describing. Once one has grasped the uniqueness of metaphor in combining both abstraction and seeing or sensing, one can begin to account for its power to enlarge and "bootstrap" thought. And since, according to Lakoff and Turner (1989), conscious knowledge is commonly understood through the metaphor "Knowing is seeing," when we see something in a new way, we know it in a new way.

   This process of abstractive seeing—of mapping our sensed experience into abstractions to create new understanding—is most vividly and systematically exploited by imaginative writers. Let me give an example from a novelist, George Dennison. In his novel, *Luisa Domic* (1985), Dennison uses metaphors to depict the metaphor-making process in all its wonder. Twelve-year-old Ida has just turned to her father on their farm and asked him to tell a visiting friend about the swallows they had seen the previous summer:

> She meant the sleek and powerful fork-tailed swallows who in varying numbers came back to our barn year after year. They were the swiftest of flyers, and all summer long, just before dark, after their hunting for insects was ended, they had

sprinted as had the ponies, hurtling round and round the house at high speed in breathtaking undulant loops.

But the memory that dwelt in Ida's mind, and that brought such a glow to her face, was really of something else. We had sat side by side on the topmost wooden stop of the unroofed front porch, in the greenest and sweetest of late summer evenings, and had watched the ponies speed by, and had watched the swallows circling the house, swooping out to the barn and back, around and around; and admiring all these things, we had fallen unaware into a bliss of contentment. I had said to her, "The swallows are like dolphins," and her face had brightened. She knew exactly what I meant. And because I saw that look of discovery on her face (she was glimpsing new uses of the process of abstraction; she was seeing another of the many ways in which accumulated experience acquired mental form and was discovering that the analytic mode could be a mode of praise), because I saw that look, I said to her, "Tell me what the dolphins and swallows and greyhounds and cheetahs and falcons have in common," and she grinned and said, "Oh, they're speedy, Dad!" And I said, "Yes, and they have in common that they make you say 'Oh' "—at which she smiled more brightly still, being well aware that she had just said "Oh!" We agreed that our ponies, delightful as they were, were not fast enough or splendid enough to be included in that company. "But they make us say 'Oh!' " she said. "We say it all the time"—and we talked of the "Oh!" of delight, or of admiration touched by love, and the "Oh!" of praise and tribute, or of admiration touched by awe.

All this was what she meant when she looked at me with that glowing face and said, "Tell him about the swallows, Dad." (pp. 39–40)

The Vividness of Metaphors: They Make You Say "Oh!"

I have cited this passage from Dennison in order to convey both the concreteness and the abstraction involved in the metaphoric process. But even more important, I want to set vibrating the idea that affect and metaphor are closely connected, that the mode of analogy can be "the mode of praise." In my view, an image-laden metaphor that is novel is usually born out of intense feeling: the need to communicate something never communicated in that way before, to make others see what you have seen, and very often to express psychological states that can only be *approximated* in words. These ineffable feeling states are either too vague, too complex, or too intense for ordinary speech. States of ecstasy or despair, and experiences of feared annihilation or mystical union all cry out for metaphors to approximate their feeling component. "My cup runneth over" is an outer equivalent for an inner psychological state of fullness and grace.

Furthermore, the very concreteness of metaphor engages us as abstractions never can. A metaphor has for us the power that a case example does: It gives flesh and blood to the abstract and theoretical. Metaphor, especially when used deliberately and unconventionally, says, "Look at me! Look *at* the word, not *through* it." Indeed, our words and our patients' words become objects of great significance.

Think of the difference, for instance, between saying "Used car salesmen are generally sneaky and untrustworthy" and "Used car salesmen are snakes." The word "snake" carries an image with surplus meaning of feelings and associations: All the associations that we have collectively and individually to snakes surge in with the image we may be seeing in our mind's eye. Is it a boa constrictor about to surround its prey, a rattlesnake slithering through the grass, a cobra raising its mysterious hood? A whole tangle of conscious and unconscious associations (including fertility, feminine wisdom, Satan as tempter, the capacity for self-transformation, as well as penises limp and erect) goes with the image, and metaphor delivers them in an economical and vivid package.

For the paradox in metaphor, as we have seen, is that the abstract is arrived at through the concrete, through the senses. What gives metaphor its *usefulness* is the possibility of bridging or generalizing so that thought can cover a larger domain than originally. But what gives metaphor its *vividness* and resonance is its connection with the world of sensed and felt experience. The source term is most often visual, since vision is our most developed sense, occupying a larger area in the cerebral cortex than all the other senses. But sometimes our metaphors are auditory (note the use of resonance above), and certainly we and our patients draw on gustatory, tactile, and even kinesthetic metaphors. We *taste* our patients' sorrow, we are *touched* by their pleasure, we often *feel* the rightness of our intuition about them. So the paradox is that the vividly sensuous becomes a vehicle for abstraction and generalization, for wider meaning, and as I shall show later, for the symbolic imagination that is so crucial to human function and so much at the heart of the process of psychotherapy.

METAPHOR AND THE ORIGIN
OF THOUGHT

The Developmental Primacy of Metaphor:
Children as Metaphorists

The capacity to analogize using concrete experience is apparent early in our life history. In research on creativity, Gardner (1982) has demonstrated that even very young children are fluent metaphor makers. But a striking point emerges from his research: These early metaphors are image metaphors, usually based on physical properties. The analogy is from one physical form to another based on perceptual similarities of the objects that are being compared. For example, one child likens an elephant's trunk and head to "a gas mask"; another sees a potato chip as "a cowboy hat"; for a third, a red balloon becomes "an apple."

Furthermore, much of the child's early metaphor-making (in the third or fourth year of life) arises from action or symbolic play. At this age, as Piaget (1954) has amply demonstrated, the child is both concrete and action oriented. Thus, a child may chew on a pencil (a cylindrical yellow object) and pretend to be eating corn (another cylindrical yellow object). Indeed, Santostefano (1988), in describing his clinical work with children, seeks to broaden the definition of metaphor to include metaphors of action and of fantasy images as well as of words. He has typically found that as the analytic work with troubled children progresses, they are more likely to use verbal metaphors than to express their metaphors nonverbally by enacting them.

In normal development, as children get older, they are less insistent that the object closely resemble what it represents in play. Because, as Piaget has demonstrated, they are less and less tied to the concrete; they can designate an object to represent a wide variety of things. But there are limits: a milk bottle, for example, can be used to represent a person, but it cannot readily be used to represent a cloud or a flower.

And sometimes the enactive component gives way to more complex physical analogies without action. One of the child subjects of Gardner and Winner (1982) described his mother's hair as "dark woods." Another thought of a jet trail as "a scar in the sky." An internal perception was likened to an external one as the sensation of feet falling asleep was compared to bubbling gingerale. And perhaps the whiff of a beginning capacity for empathy can be sniffed in one child's comparison of a flashlight battery to "a sleeping bag all rolled up and ready to go to a friend's house" (p. 93).

So the rule for most early metaphors, during the preschool years, seems to be that comparison across domains is based on perceptual resemblance, similarity in action, or both. Gardner and Winner (1982) say, "Virtually never have we encountered [among children of that age] a figure of speech that bears psychological connotations" (p. 99). They also note that many metaphors of children are simply indecipherable because they are so idiosyncratic and private.

Another important finding of this research is that the metaphor-making capacity seems to wane when the child enters school and throughout the elementary school years. This finding fits with research on children's drawings, which become less imaginative and more literal when the child enters school. In general, this is a time of industriousness and rule-boundedness. We know from the work of Piaget (1951, 1955) that children in elementary school regard rules as sacrosanct and demand rigid adherence to them. Children do not stop making metaphors altogether, but they increasingly learn to use the more conventional, less idiosyncratic metaphors of the wider culture. These are the kinds of metaphors we all use so automatically that we no longer consciously register them as metaphors (e.g., "I see what you mean," "She put me down," etc.) Once in school, the child uses metaphors that are less vivid, less idiosyncratic, less imagistic; he or she has learned the rules of everyday speech, whose metaphors are subtly but indispensably woven into the fabric of discourse.

Adolescence brings both an upsurge of sexual impulse, and the cognitive freedom to hypothesize and to make reasoned guesses about the formal properties of objects, events, and even propositions. It is then that young people begin to see the connections between physical and emotional states, and to use metaphors intentionally to link the abstract and the concrete.

Primary Process Thinking and Metaphor: Freud's Distinctions

We have seen how children use figurative language quite naturally. There are grounds for believing that the imagistic symbolic mode goes back to the first "thought" of infancy. In what many regard as his most seminal contribution, Freud (1911) distinguished two modes of thought—the primary process and the secondary process. The primary process is the first mental process the infant relies on; it is hallucinatory and wishfulfilling, and characterizes dreams and psychosis as well as other manifestations of the unconscious. Freud (1911) describes the primary process as drive-directed, timeless, and contradictionless, permitting opposites to be maintained simultaneously. He also tells us that it is mostly pictorial or imagistic rather than verbal, and—to use his hydraulic metaphor—fluid in its energy disposition. Condensation and displacement are its primary modes of operation. So, in a dream, one image can "stand for" many things simultaneously: A boat can be the domineering mother in full sail, as well as the ego or directed part of the dreamer's personality, and the night sea journey of psychotherapy itself. The substitutability of one image for another is its guiding principle; hence, metaphor is deeply rooted in the primary process.

In Freud's view, the secondary process, by contrast, is reality-oriented, rather than drive-oriented, with fixed cathexes of energy. Words are used denotatively rather than connotatively: The meaning is narrowed down as precisely as possible, and one statement follows from another by discursive logic. Something cannot be itself and not-itself at the same time. For Freud, this was presumably the mode of rational thought and—in its most pristine form—the mode of science. He believed that secondary process was the hallmark of ego rather than id: Its pursuit was to be fostered, its domain expanded.

What Freud did not sufficiently emphasize is that the primary process is not simply the mode of infantile wishes, dreams, conversion symptoms, and hallucinations. It is also the mode of the imaginal and, therefore, of art—of poetry and literature. There are some who hold with Johnson (1988) that even this distinction is meaningless since so-called rationality draws heavily on images and metaphors, so that reason and imagination can never be separated. This may be true in an ultimate way, but I myself believe that some of the distinction is worth preserving. Perhaps it is most useful to think of primary process and secondary process not as dichotomous but as continuous. At one end of the continuum are dreams and at the other end is mathematical reasoning. And in between is thinking that reflects both wish-fulfillment and objectivity, the proportions depending on how close it is to either end.

If we think of the two processes this way, we may be able to avoid the disjunction seemingly implied in Freud's primary process.[1] Metaphor can help us here. Secondary process thought in its purest form is linear: If you want to get from point 1 to point 4, you have to pass through points 2 and 3 in that order along a straight line. I say "in its purest form" because I agree with Bruner (1986) that most of our thinking is drenched in affect; it requires a special act of will to pursue objective, abstract thought.

Primary process thinking is weblike: If you touch point 1, a node in the web, you will see connections to other points on the web, some far distant. If you pluck one point on the web, the entire web will tremble and resonate. In thinking of these two processes as continuous rather than as dichotomous, we are perhaps thinking of how a web could gradually be transformed in shape to become more linear.

In speaking of the primary process end of the continuum, I have used the metaphor of resonance intentionally because it takes us into the domain of music—of harp strings and tuning forks. And similarity on the basis of sound is one of the characteristics that Freud (1911) clearly recognized as a property of unconscious logic. Slips of the tongue and puns have a logic of their own, and in altered states of consciousness, when the ego is less active, these sound-substitutions are more obvious. Thus, Jung in his early work with the word association experiment (Jung & Riklin, 1973) found that when attention wavered, that is, when the subjects grew fatigued over long series of words, they gave more of what we call "clang" associations—that is, homonyms or associations based on sound.

In Freud's study of the "Rat Man" (1909), we see how someone with an obsessional neurosis is plagued by phonetic associations that tap into his major complex. The patient was obsessed with the fear of being attacked by rats (*Ratten*). In the course of his analysis, as described by Kugler (1982), it became clear that

> each of the patient's unresolved conflicts was related phoneti-
> cally to the sound-pattern [rat]. The man was disturbed over
> the installments ("*Raten*") he had made on his father's gam-
> bling ("*Spielratte*") debts. He also had never recovered from
> the early death of his sister, *Rita*, nor could he decided whether
> or not to marry ("*heiraten*") at the courthouse ("*Rathaus*). In
> the phonic resonance of his patient's words, Freud discovered a
> psychic logic. (p. 67)[2]

In emphasizing the sound-and-image properties of the primary process, I am calling attention to the concreteness of figurative language and its derivation from something deep and primary within us, an early mode of functioning that is available to "dreamers, poets, and madmen" but very different in the way it is used by poets—and by most patients—than by dreamers and those who are awash in the primary process.

A Non-Pathologizing View of Primary Process: Differences between the Dreaming and the Waking Imagination

I have already noted one of Freud's most seminal contributions: his distinction between the primary and the secondary processes of thinking and his explication of how in the primary process, various images, impulses, and "clang" association are combined to produce a unique language of the unconscious. By applying this language to dreams, slips of the tongue, and jokes, he immensely widened our sense of the outcroppings of the unconscious in daily—and nightly—life.

But Freud's distinction carried with it a biased judgment with undue pathologizing of the unconscious. For Freud, the goal is to translate the imagistic impulse language of the unconscious into the syntactic, discursive logic of the ego. This puts a heavy freight on the voice of science and 19th-century rationalism while tending to regard the products of the unconscious as pathological.

One of the most vocal dissenters from Freud's pejorative view is Charles Rycroft, a British psychoanalyst of the so-called Independent School. Rycroft withdrew from the British psychoanalytic association on a number of grounds, but mainly because he felt the psychoanalytic establishment took too reductive a view of symbolization.

In *The Innocence of Dreams*, Rycroft (1979) takes issue with the traditional psychoanalytic view espoused by Ernest Jones and others that symbols are fixed in a one-to-one way ("cup," for example, always and only equals "vagina") and that they are necessarily the expression of repressed primitive impulses. He believes that this view gives the primary process a regressive and pathological cast, which is wrong-headed in general and particularly askew in the case of the artist. Actually, Freud was very responsive to imaginative literature, and he repeatedly said that his ancestors in the discovery of the unconscious were poets and philosophers rather than doctors and scientists. And at the same time, he was uneasy about accounting for the origins or the power of art. Perhaps he had the sense that "sublimation" was not adequate to the explanatory task, for in his essay on Dostoevsky and parricide, he wrote, "Before the problem of the creative artist analysis must, alas, lay down its arms" (quoted in Rycroft, 1979, p. 39). Rycroft goes on to say that the artist only becomes a "problem" if the imagination is thought to be allied to dreams, which Freud himself equated with symptoms.

Perhaps it will help at this point, using Rycroft as guide, to explore the difference between the dream image and the metaphoric image.

DREAM IMAGE VERSUS METAPHORIC IMAGE

Displacement is the process that underlies symbol formation and figures of speech, both in dreams and in waking life. Or, as Rycroft (1979) puts it more felicitously, "Symbolization is a general capacity and propensity which creates metaphors when used con-sciously and dream-images when occurring while dreaming" (p. 75). Further, the imagery in the dream "lacks as yet the meaning that will turn it into metaphor," as though it is "a thought that has yet to acquire the author who will give it metaphorical meaning" (p. 71).

In therapy, the patient reporting a dream is the author through his or her associations, and the therapist becomes a kind of col-laborator through his or her interpretations. This view echoes Aristo-tle's view that the best interpreter of dreams is the person who can best grasp similarities, that is, a master of metaphor.

Rycroft (1979) sees dreaming essentially as involuntary imag-inative activity. Dreams have a surreal form not because of an attempt to censor and disguise but because of the very nature of dreaming: First of all, dreaming is private, and hence dreams need not make sense to a wider audience; and second, the higher cortical processes are asleep. Both these circumstances cause dreamers to "present their imaginings to themselves not in the discursive language they use to convey meanings to others but in non-discursive symbolism" (p. 46).

Unlike factual or scientific statements in which the terms are operationally defined so that each term has one clear meaning, dreams, like novels and poems, have manifold meanings; the dream imagination unites and condenses a number of images with remarkable brevity. This is why a paraphrase will be much longer than the poem it summarizes and why a dream interpretation may be longer than the experienced dream.

The dreaming imagination and the waking imagination, says Rycroft, are alike in creating new products by combining and con-densing images and ideas. Both do this in a not altogether "willed" way. This is very clear for dreams. But it is also true to a lesser extent for fantasies and daydreams, which appear to "happen" to the subject, often in a state of diffuse consciousness—in hypnogogic states, rever-ies, and dissociations from ordinary conscious effort. (The literature on creativity teems with creative moments occurring through dreams or on long train journeys when the attention of the artist or scientist is free-floating rather than narrowly task-oriented.)

A crucial difference between dreams and daydreams, however, is that in the waking imagination the critical, rational, "editing" forces that determine the selection of images are also operating.

Dreams, Rycroft (1979) tells us, are not only involuntary poetry but incomplete poetry because they are unedited: "They more often resemble someone who is groping for the appropriate metaphor than someone who has found it" (p. 165).

And, in terms that sound rather Jungian, Rycroft asserts that what creates such products—both dream images and metaphors—is not the "I" or ego but "some wider, less personal self to which the 'I' must yield . . . [and] by which our personal, egotistical self is lived" (p. 19). This "It" (Freud's *Das Es*, the id) is what "dreams us," what sends us messages. Although he disagrees with much in Jung, Rycroft seems to agree with him that "The dream is a mysterious message from our night aspect" (p. 32).

The primary process occurs in dreaming by the simple act of falling asleep; it manifests in our waking life in moments of heightened or lowered consciousness, often in a state of reverie. Rycroft compares this state to what Keats described as a prerequisite to writing poetry: a condition of "negative capability"—the faculty of allowing oneself to remain in a state of "uncertainties, mysteries, doubts, without any irritable reaching after fact and reason."

The state of mind of Keats's ideal poet is not unlike the "evenly suspended attention" recommended to analysts by Freud. It is a state that appears to be midway between waking and dreaming. In delineating the two principles of mental functioning what Freud did not sufficiently distinguish perhaps was that third thing—*the waking imagination*—which produces fantasies, daydreams, and metaphors. It partakes of both primary and secondary process but forms a new synthesis. Drawing on the unconscious for images, impulses, and motives, it applies conscious control to the ordering and arranging of them. Jung (1916) had a sense of this more clearly than any other psychologist of his day when he described the process of "active imagination." This was a deliberate attempt to work with the mysterious or ego-alien aspects of dreams or fantasy images and to set them in deliberate dialogue with the conscious attitude so that out of this work some new synthesis—a third thing—would be born.

This process itself takes the form that metaphor takes. You will remember the "formula" for constructing metaphor: Map aspects of an experienced source domain into an abstract target domain, such that a new concept emerges. The analogy, that "third thing," is what is novel, what has not been put together quite that way before. Jung (1921) stresses that to be a symbol, rather than a sign, the analogy must point to some hitherto unknown bit of psychic reality.

I would like through case material to show what I observe constantly in my clinical work: how a patient reverts to metaphor to express such psychic reality during a time of great emotion and how its use conveys psychological possibility that ordinary language cannot reveal.

THE AFFECTIVE PRIMACY OF METAPHOR: CASE EXAMPLES

I do not intend to suggest that every time a patient or a therapist uses a metaphor, deep wells of affect are being plumbed. There are times when the affect is hard to reach, especially in conventional or automatic metaphors (see Chapter 3). And there are times when metaphor is used defensively as a way to avoid affect through indirection (see Chapter 5). But most often I have found that figurative language springs from strong affect that cannot be conveyed in any other way. That is why if we stay with the metaphor—nurturing it and allowing it to expand—we can help deepen our patients' responses to it.

Some authors (e.g., Barlow et al., 1977) relate the affect-producing potential of metaphor to insight. The "aha" experience of seeing a connection where there had hitherto been disjunction is emotionally gratifying. It may be that when a patient employs a metaphor knowingly, he or she is motivated by strong feeling to begin with, and the new knowledge that accompanies the analogy is thereby also charged with affect. And we know that the only insights that are usable are affectively realized truths.

Metaphor flows from affect because it usually represents the need to articulate a pressing inner experience of oneself and of one's internalized objects. It typically arises when feelings are high and when ordinary words do not seem strong enough or precise enough to convey the experience.

Scott S., a man in his early thirties has been struggling for some while with me in the transference and internally with the Negative

Mother. One day, as he gets closer to termination, and begins to talk about that as a possibility, he says. "I feel I'm a butterfly."

My antennae (to use a similar metaphor) go up, as they do whenever a figure of speech, particularly one representing the self, is introduced. If my train of thought, largely subverbal and preconscious, were to be made conscious, it would go something like this: "He's onto something here. A butterfly?" And I would see some image, probably in this case a Monarch butterfly, alighting and opening and shutting its wings, then flying off.

The *seeing* is a crucial part of my response; I am attempting to see what the patient sees. My initial image—to be corrected by what he says next—depends on my own associative net. I see a Monarch butterfly, and at an almost subliminal level, I wonder what aspect of this butterfly he will focus on—the brilliance of color, the rapidity of flight, or the movement in repose.

He shifts the image slightly so that I now have a clearer intuition about what he means: "A butterfly halfway out of the pupa case." Now the image has been refined, and its coloration has changed. I see a butterfly emerging from its cocoon; now the associations that this image touches off in me are those of birth (infants emerging from the birth canal) and of transformation (one stage in the life cycle melding into another). And I wonder: Is this an easy or painful "birth"? Is the emphasis on liberation and freedom, or on loss?

"I am that butterfly halfway out of the pupa. Down to here" (He gestures toward his midsection).

And then without prompting from me, partly because he has had experiences in the past of our being on the same figurative wavelength, he produces his own associative memory:

My son's nursery school class collected caterpillars and watched them grow into butterflies. I remember going into the classroom and being bowled over by the sight of the pupa case. I guess I hadn't expected anything so beautiful . . . It was pale green, iridescent where the light hit it. You could imagine a butterfly wanting to stay in it forever.

(He might, I thought, have wanted to stay with his mother forever, or to stay with me in the safe container of this therapy forever.)

I was there when the butterfly emerged, and it was enormously exciting, but my son asked a question that I thought was profound: He said, "Does the caterpillar know it will become a butterfly, and does the butterfly know it's been a caterpillar?"

Scott may not have been aware of it, but he was reflecting a long tradition of speculation about butterflies. Synchronistically, while working on this chapter, I was pointed by a colleague to an essay on metaphor by the poet Howard Nemerov (1985). In this piece Nemerov cites three examples of the caterpillar-into-butterfly motif that so tantalized my patient and his small son: Dante in *The Divine Comedy* writes:

> *Noi siam vermi, nati a formar*
> *L'angelica farfalla.*
>
> We are caterpillars, born to become
> The angelic butterfly.

Ophelia, in *Hamlet*, says musingly, "We know what we are but not what we may become." And Marshall McLuhan offers a cartoon of a caterpillar, looking at a butterfly, and saying, "Waal, you'll never catch me in one of those durn things."

My patient, in producing this memory, was talking about the ineffable mystery of change and transformation. He used this symbolic form to talk metaphorically about his own growth and development in the therapeutic process. I did not feel called upon to get him to expand the metaphor or even to associate further to it; this far along, he could do most of his own work. I simply shared his wonder at the mysteriousness of his own transformation, and his concern about what it would be like to leave the pupa-case of this therapy.

Another case example: Marie C., an illustrator in her early 30s, had continued to live out the myth of her working-class family that she as a child was "out to lunch" because she spent so much time in fantasy play. In fact, she is a person of clear and definite tastes and ambitions. She has been much more successful in her work and her marriage than her mother was. When Marie was 11, she had fallen and suffered severe pain in her arm and shoulder. Her mother, a religious fundamentalist, treated her with aspirin and the invocation to pray to maintain her divine image. Finally, the pain got so acute and the swelling so severe, she had to be taken to a hospital emergency room for treatment. As Marie recalled the senseless suffering she had had to endure, she allowed herself to feel outrage toward her mother for the first time in her life. It became clear to me and through me to her, that her mother was the one who had been "out to lunch," denying the shadow aspects of her own life. Much of the work Marie and I did together had to do with this "possession" by her maternal introject, which forced her to take her mother's view (or, more correctly, her idea of her mother's view) of herself.

As she began to see the disparities and the nature of this largely self-imposed bondage, and to accept the painfulness of her negative feelings toward her mother, she produced a metaphor that signaled her entry into a new territory of selfhood:

My mother has no tolerance for her own dark side; it was always put outside of herself—onto Satan or nonbelievers. She was untainted—like a pure white canvas. But if I think of my life as a painting, it has all kinds of colors. [She said this with passion in her voice, her hands gesturing to trace in the air the shape of a canvas]. And I believe that every day we add to this painting, and it's very complex: it's got dark colors, light colors—what those Renaissance guys called chiaroscuro—*it's varied and rich, a whole* paletteful *of colors. And the dark is what highlights the bright.*

Another patient, Sharon P., trying to convey to me her experience of feeling overwhelmed by the demands of others, and having insufficient boundaries or defenses to withstand any imperious request, especially from a man, said, "I can't find the words, but I could draw it, if I could draw, because the feeling is so clear to me, and so overwhelming." When I asked what she would draw if she could, she said:

I would draw sea and sand, and I am the sand. When the sea pounds at the sand, it can't resist. It simply gets sucked up and out. I wonder how something as formless and light as sand can resist the pounding and pull of the surf? That frightens me.

As I listen to Sharon, her image affects me both emotionally and cognitively. I can now feel more truly how overwhelmed and powerless she feels. And I begin to associate privately and somewhat dreamily to seawalls and breakwaters—some way we can work together to help her build some ego boundaries.

In talking of affect, I am irresistibly drawn to musical analogies. We can think of metaphor as reflecting not so much the words as the music of experience. Finding the right metaphor is, in my experience, like coming on a new melody and feeling it was there for you all the time waiting to be heard. I had an experience of this sort the first time I heard Mozart's "*Ruhe sanft, mein holdes leben*" from *Zaide*; it seemed to me that the song had been there from the beginning of time and that Mozart had not invented it so much as discovered it.

An apt metaphor has the same inevitability. The musical metaphor is not accidental. Music and feeling have always been connected in our minds, and, indeed, Langer (1948) held that music was a vehicle that expressed nuances of feelings in a formal way. I believe that the musical analogy underlies the therapeutic process at its heart, and I shall expand this analogy in the final chapter.

Not only does metaphor arise from strong feelings, it also generates such feelings. And when a patient's metaphor is really taken in by the therapist, it leads to the sense that one has communicated a bit of oneself to the other and that that bit of self has been held and valued. In this way, it deepens the communicative well from which patient and therapist jointly draw.

Metaphor generates affect in another, equally important way. In successfully conjuring up the "third thing" via a linking of two domains, the patient or therapist has performed a synthesizing operation. I maintain that whenever an integration takes place—whether on a large scale, which happens rarely, or on a small local scale, which happens fairly regularly in therapy—the person making the connection feels a complex set of emotions reflecting psychological development at several levels: At the level of oedipal and postoedipal development, the patient experiences a sense of mastery—of actively joining and bringing together—that releases pride in one's product ("Mommy, look what I made!") At the same time, in the same person, earlier preoedipal and even preverbal experiences are evoked as well. Not only is the metaphor-maker an active joiner and linker, but he or she is also a passive experiencer of such joinings; it is as though bits of the self get linked together and that experience partakes of our earliest fusions (being held in the womb, being held by a parent). Thus it can produce blissful feelings of oneness (what Freud [1929] called the "oceanic feeling") as well as the pride of mastery.

CONCLUSION

Our journey in this chapter has taken us across a wide terrain. I have moved in a spiral rather than a straight line to touch on topics and then circle back to them. Perhaps a better metaphor than the spiral or circle is the one I suggested at the outset—the web. The idea of "primacy" is the central node in this web, with strands radiating out and back. "Primary" means earlier in time, deeper in level, and greater in importance. I have talked about the primacy of metaphor in the development of thought and as the cornerstone of both poetic and everyday discourse: the basic way we increase our understanding. The primary process draws on the processes of condensation and combination that metaphor uses. This protothought continues beyond infancy to enter not only into dreams but also, in a more voluntary way, into daydreams and fantasies. The primacy of this analogy-making in human cognition can be seen from readiness of very young children to link disparate items through perceptual likeness. Furthermore, we have seen that metaphor has a primacy in affective as well as cognitive terms.

Since metaphor is also, of course, the stuff of poetry, we find that at the most advanced as well as the most "primitive" reaches of the imagination, this process of creating new wholes through analogy is at work. Poets are supremely skilled in this domain. But we all have a latent poet within us, and our patients will produce such poetry if we will only listen and provide a fostering atmosphere.

The difference in quality between poets' (or patients') and dreamers' use of primary process depends on the deliberateness and secondary revision by the ego. This interplay between the imaging unconscious and the structuring conscious suggests a similarity to what Jung (1916) called the "transcendent function." I have depicted the metaphoric imagination as a way to reach the unknown, the inner states that beggar description. These states of strong affect demand the heightened and vivid language that calls attention to them by its sensory qualities and its difference from ordinary speech.

Since metaphor links domains and grows out of and yields strong feelings, it becomes a natural vehicle for therapeutic work. It may not be "the royal road," but it is certainly a major thoroughfare to the unconscious.

I will talk more about working clinically with metaphor in later chapters. Here I want simply to stress the importance of pricking up our ears and opening our third eye in response to metaphors, for surely these can be the signal that (to paraphrase Shakespeare) "something fateful this way comes."

NOTES

1. I say "seemingly" because at times Freud expressed what later writers regard as a more fruitful way to think of primary process, namely as having a dialectical, rather than a linear, relationship to secondary process. Thus, Loewald (1988), citing Freud's essay on Leonardo, writes:

We tend to think automatically of transmutation from lower to higher levels as a form of progression from coarse, crude states or processes to more refined, advanced ones. In the . . . Leonardo study Freud suggests a different vista: The "lowest" and "highest" are enveloped as one within an original unitary experience; one *is* the other, and later they can stand for one another, the deity a symbol of the living sexual body . . . there is a symbolic *linkage* which constitutes what we call meaning. (p. 13)

Loewald adds that in emphasizing the hidden linkage between what is sublimated or differentiated through secondary process and what is defended against, "psychoanalysis reveals the inextricable bond of primary and secondary process" (p. 13).

2. In *The Alchemy of Discourse: An Archetypal Approach to Language*, Kugler (1982), a Jungian analyst, assumes "a poetic and mythological basis of mind" (p. 13). Kugler holds with Jung that words whose meanings are related to the same archetypal image have similar sounds. Jung noted the phonetic equivalents in many languages between "mother" (German, "mar," French "mère") and the word for sea (Lat. "Mare," G. "Meer," F. "mer") and said that although these similarities were etymologically accidental, they might point back to "the great primordial image of the mother who was once our only world and later became the symbol of the whole world" (quoted in Kugler, p.

26). Kugler points to the concurrence in several languages of flowers and violence or sexual violation (violet/violate; de-flowering; carnation, reincarnation, carnage, carnal). Such similarities are found not only in English but in other languages (German, French, Hungarian). He feels they reflect the archetypal theme of the rape of Persephone, who is gathering flowers when the earth opens up and Hades plucks her to the underworld to consummate their marriage by force. Kugler says words become phonetically equated because they once shared an archetypal image-meaning: "Perhaps the reason dreamers, poets, and madmen display such an uncanny sense of the depth of the imagination is that their perceptual systems—like those of the oral tellers of myths—are tuned to the invariant archetypal structures of sound and image" (p. 28). It would be useful to see if these findings also hold across *non*-Indo-European languages.

CHAPTER 2

The Bodily Matrix of Metaphor

The shapes and relations and names of objects [of desire] are unknown to the infant's mind. Food it knows, but not the source of food, beyond the mere touch and vague form of the mother's breast. . . . Everything soft is a mother; everything that meets his reach is food. Being dropped, even into bed, is terror itself—the first definite form of insecurity, even of death (all our lives we speak of misfortune as a "fall": we fall into the enemy's hands, fall from grace, fall upon hard times).

SUSANNE LANGER, Philosophy in a New Key

Metaphor making, we have seen, is the primary quality of all new language and of the unconscious. It draws on our earliest experiences, which are experiences of the body. Metaphor, the basic way of increasing our understanding, uses body experience as the vehicle through which it reaches out to nonbodily experience, just as an artist uses physical media—clay, paint, metal, stone—to evoke nonphysical ideas, visions, or states. And because being embodied is our primary and most continuous experience, it is no wonder that when we speak of walls and fences, prisons and sanctuaries, in and out, armor and wounds, barriers and the rupturing of barriers, our primary referent is our own bodily experience.

This chapter begins with an impressionistic description of body image and then turns to some speculations on body imagery and affect, which will lead to a consideration of a seminal article on metaphor and bodily experience. I will then illustrate through a case example the similarities and differences between symptom and metaphor. Finally, I will show how true insight is experienced in and through the body.

A MEDITATION ON THE BODY

The most "real" thing about us from the beginning is our embodiedness. Our first perceptions *in utero* are of visceral sensations, and we are constantly getting feedback of our boundedness—the kinesthetic knowledge that we have limbs that move and stretch and cramp and reach. Something in our chest races, slows, pounds, skips beats; something up there clenches when danger approaches. Something "down there" roils when we are afraid. And we can feel real products streaming out of our openings—saliva, urine, sweat, feces—that are objects first of wonder, later often of distaste.

As embodied creatures, we feel the inhaling and exhaling of our breath, the temperature of the air on our skin, the touch that is bruising or caressing. Sensations in the gut tell us that we are achingly empty, deliciously full, or uncomfortably bloated. From inside, our muscle sense tells us whether the body is anchored or falling, being snuggled or smothered, flailing or resting easy.

In *The Ego and the Id,* Freud (1923) held that the ego was "first and foremost a body ego," which makes itself on body experiences. He wrote:

> A person's own body, and above all its surface, is a place from which both external and internal perceptions may spring. It is *seen* like any other object, but to the touch it yields two kinds of sensations, one of which may be equivalent to an internal perception. Psychophysiology has fully discussed the manner in which a person's own body attains its special position among other objects in the world of perception. (p. 15)

Indeed, all of our more sophisticated experiences of me and not-me come originally from the matrix of bodily experience. They originate from what is in and what is out: what we take in with the eyes, what we devour with the mouth, what we suck into us, hold onto with the gut, or expel easily or effortfully.

A baby in a crib twirls its hand and watches it in wonder. Is it she or not-she? At this point, perhaps, it does not matter. This small, curvy twisting object is both kinesthetically felt from inside and experienced as the external object of curiosity, looking, and watching that defines a relationship with the world.

High and low were originally based on what needs to be looked at with the head raised and what needs to be looked at with the head lowered. As children, we literally looked up to our parents, the avatars of the divine, and we looked down to small animals, worms, flowers, insects, the earth.

Warm and cold, which later become psychological attributes of persons, were originally registered through and in the body, with its chills, fevers, or experiences of blissful warmth. Similarly, hard and soft were first felt by each of us as what our bodies reposed on, whether cradle or crib or the breasts of caretakers.

All our later feelings of bliss and dejection have their roots in the nursery and in the body. Body experiences are so peremptory that they carry with them their own seal of acceptance as "the real." And because these experiences are so primal and irrefutable, so literally palpable, they become the sources of our most crucial metaphors: the concrete in terms of which the abstract is presented. Thus, moments of merging with a loving caregiver, a bodily ecstasy, are the early physical basis for later states of bliss, whether they be intimate union with a partner or ecstatic religious states.

We can understand how basic this body sense is to the survival of the ego when we study the effects of its aberrations. Freud (1923) says that pain seems to be a vehicle for experiencing our bodies, and "the way we gain a knowledge of our organs during painful illnesses is perhaps a model of the way by which in general we arrive at the idea of our body" (pp. 25–26). What Freud does not talk about is how disturbances of the experience of the body—when one of its parts looms above all others or fails to register at all—are enormously distressing to the ego. It leads to the distortion and dis-ease W. H. Auden referred to in his poem "Surgical Ward," in which a wounded person becomes his wounded part: Those of us who are healthy cannot imagine what it means, for example, to "become a foot." Even more traumatic are disturbances in which a taken-for-granted part fails to preserve not only its function but its customary registration: Oliver Sacks (1984), in describing the accident that left him with the sight and touch of his own leg but without its registration in his central nervous system (and hence without any feel of it at all), writes:

> The leg had vanished, taking its "past" away with it. I could no longer remember how I had ever walked and climbed. I felt

inconceivably cut off from the person who had walked and run, and climbed just five days before. There was only a "formal" continuity between us. There was a gap—an absolute gap— between then and now; and in that gap, into the void, the former "I" had vanished—the "I" who could thoughtlessly stand, run and walk, who was totally and thoughtlessly sure of his body, who couldn't conceive how doubts about it could possibly arise. . . . Into the gap, that void, outside space and time, the reality and possibilities of the leg had passed, and disappeared. . . . my own leg had vanished "into the blue." ' . . . it had vanished from space and time—vanished taking its space-and-time with it. (pp. 85–86)

Sacks has described an extreme occurrence that is not within the experience of most of us or our patients. Yet such extreme states amplify what we often feel in lesser form—the utter primacy of the body sensations both in time and in our experience. What is real is what is felt with and through the body. Thus, it is no wonder that these experiences become the basic currency of metaphors of less tangible states of affect.

THE PRIMACY AND SPECIALNESS OF BODY EXPERIENCE

In contrast to the affect-tinged descriptions of body I have given above, consider this more scientific view of Fisher (1970):

The experienced body is a world within a world. It is a complexly shaped and yet bilaterally symmetrically simplified object which has spatial and geographical features second to none in their diversity. . . . [T]he body possesses an interior which, though hidden from others and therefore socially invisible continues to be evident to oneself with vivid intensity. One knows one's body from the inside, although the insides of other opaque objects are almost never perceivable. (p. 567)

One thing that makes the body peculiar in our experience is that is it the only opaque object one senses from the inside as well as the outside.

— 27 —

In addition, the body is equated with the self more than any other object is. When the infant achieves personhood, he or she has a personal pattern of psychosomatic life. Winnicott (1960) calls it "psyche indwelling in soma." The body serves as a framework for all our sensory experience in giving us steady feedback about its changes. Fisher (1970) says that the concept of "self" is often expressed in terms of bodily sensation (e.g., I feel light or heavy or down or queasy, etc.). Furthermore, we locate the "self" within our body and often experience it as coterminous with the body. It is hard to imagine a disembodied self.

Fisher and Cleveland (1968), in their useful review of depth psychologies and the body, point out that the major depth psychologists have recognized the centrality of body in their explorations of the psyche. Body experience of zones and modes is, of course, the cornerstone of Freud's system, summed up in his famous dictum (1923) that "the ego is first and foremost a body ego." Freud believed that the early development of the ego occurred as the child learned to organize sensations from the body surface and to use those sensations to distinguish between self and not-self, or body and outside world. Fenichel (cited in Fisher & Cleveland, 1968) expanded on that point: From the perception of an "inside something"—a tension—the baby gradually learns that there is something—an "outside something"—that will quiet that tension:

> One's own body becomes something apart from the rest of the world, and thus the discerning of self from nonself is made possible. The sum of the mental representations of the body and its organs, the so-called body image, constitutes the idea of I and is of basic importance for the formation of the ego. (p. 42)

Indeed, Freud's entire developmental psychology was a psychology of bodily zones and modes, of condensations and displacements in which the body served as one extensive metaphor system: openings are equated (vagina = mouth); parts that project out are equated (nose = upward displacement of penis); functions are substitutable (looking is a form of incorporation).

Other depth psychologists, according to Fisher and Cleveland, have concentrated on the need to form protective boundaries. Thus,

Reich emphasized the inhibition that leads people to develop the muscular rigidity that he called "character armor." Rank thought of the vessel or container as the basic prototype of the body, originating first, perhaps, as a maternal symbol and then as a representation of the child (and we know that when children first draw the body, they draw a circle with appendages protruding from it).

Jung, too, emphasized the idea of the protective container first in terms of the maternal figure and then in terms of the mandala. The mandala is the magic circle that is found in cultures all over the world—essentially a symbol for the integrated Self. [Indeed, in his own circular tower at Bollingen, as I have noted (Siegelman, 1987), Jung honored both the "maternal hearth" and the integrated psyche.]

A follower of Jung, Gerhard Adler, gave this mandala form a specific body-image referent. Adler found that mandalas were common features in the drawings of disintegrating patients trying to reconstitute. He describes the body/mandala relationship as follows (Adler, 1951):

> An intuitive interpretation may say that the first ego experience of the baby is bound up with its skin, and that playing with its own body, it learns its demarcation from the surrounding world. It is as though the skin, the "four walls" or "circle" of the body formed a magic circle, a sort of "primordial mandala," marking off an "ego" sphere and a "non-ego" sphere, and in which the ego experiences itself sensorially. (p. 98)

Our sensations from within this magic circle of the body give us our basic system of demarcating space. Our objective sense of space seems to have evolved from the subjective experience of right–left, in front of–behind, up–down. And we know from the research of Erik Erikson (1968) on the play constructions of young boys and girls that anatomical differences are reflected in children's use of structures: Most of the girls built houses, inner spaces with ingress from the outside; the boys tended to build towers and streets (emphasizing erectile, thrusting structures or pathways to motility). Erikson perceives these constructions as reflecting anatomical differences that have been absorbed into overall body images: The external genital of the male is erectile and mobile; the external organ of the female surrounds an opening, a place of access leading to an inner space.

THE CONTAINER SCHEMA

This experience of the body as a container has important metaphoric consequences. Or, to say the same thing in the terminology of linguist George Lakoff (1987), the kinesthetic schema of "the container" leads to a number of "metaphoric entailments." "Kinesthetic schemata" represent the union of bodily experience and images that occur in everyday life. These schemata structure our experience from the beginning. Long before we have the words for up or down, we experience our vertical or horizontal orientation; we experience our body made up of parts within a whole, of being full (satiated) or empty (hungry). These experiences form the later base for our much more sophisticated metaphorical extensions of them, as when we talk about the central core of a theory and its peripheral postulates; the sense of psychological depletion or satiation in relationships (where literal food becomes replaced by psychological nourishment); and the experience of being contained versus uncontained, bounded versus unbounded.

Johnson (1987) has written that when we employ metaphor "we make use of patterns that obtain in our physical experience to organize our understanding" (p. xv). He notes that:

> We human beings have bodies. We are *"rational* animals," but we are also "rational *animals,"* which means that our rationality is embodied. The centrality of human embodiment directly influences what and how things can be meaningful for us . . . (p. xix)

Of all our kinesthetic schemata, Lakoff (1987) says, the container is perhaps the most basic, giving rise to a bounded inner space that is differentiated from what is outside. This distinction comes to shape our sense of what others have called the "me" and the "not-me." Later, we extend this schema to the perceptual world (in and out of sight), to the psychological world (in and out of moods or feeling states), and to the interpersonal world (in and out of relationships). The container schema—with things being in or out—begins with the bodily experience of ingesting and excreting air and food. Breathing in and out is our most regular and constant physical activity, a persistent subliminal reminder that our lives consist of taking in and letting out.

In showing how a "conceptual logic" grows out of this early preverbal bodily schema, Lakoff (1987) takes one affect—anger—and traces its metaphoric expressions in terms of the container. Anger is frequently spoken of metaphorically as heat. There is good ground in both experience and physiology for this metaphor: When we get angry, our pulse rate increases, our blood pressure rises, and we feel flushed and hot. Heat in a container under pressure gives us a number of ways we have learned to speak of the experience of anger: Anger, like hot fluids in a container, pushes up. One's gorge "rises," one goes into a "towering" rage, anger "wells up." Anger, like hot fluid, produces steam (we talk of fuming or blowing off steam); we can add the metaphors of cookery that also reflect heat in a container: seething, stewing, or simmering with anger, one's blood boiling. Anger, like hot fluids, produces pressure on the container: One can no longer contain one's anger, one is ready to burst with it. If intense enough, it threatens to destroy the container (we speak of blowing one's stack or hitting the ceiling).

Lakoff (1987) regards metaphor as a crucial vehicle for apprehending the many "domains of experience that do not have a preconceptual structure of their own" (p. 303). Surely, one of the domains that is most like this is the realm of strong affects such as terror, anger, depression, and bliss. These affects originally had their base in body-states, and we often use the language of the body in reconstructing them.

BODY EXPERIENCE AS THE ROOT OF PSYCHOLOGICAL METAPHORS

Our body experience shapes our orientation in space and our sense of openness versus enclosedness. It also becomes the matrix and metaphoric equivalent for *psychological*—that is, affective—states. This should not be surprising because our earliest relationships occur with and through the body. The child's early identity is a body identity, and he or she experiences adults as reacting to the cues he or she gives them about bodily sensations. At first, this is through sensation-dominated experience on the surface of the skin. In discussing this earliest mode of being, which he calls the "autistic-contiguous position," Ogden (1989) draws on work by Bick, Tustin, and others to assert that "In [this] mode, it is experiences of sensation, particularly at the skin surface, that are the principal media for the creation of psychological meaning and the rudiments of the experience of the self" (p. 52).

Later, specific body parts readily become symbolized and metaphorized. In a kind of twist of conventional Freudian wisdom, Lacan (1977) holds that the phallus is *itself* a symbol—a symbol of motility and power. And we know how susceptible the body is to symbolic distortion. Fisher and Cleveland (1968) cite the example of a man who perceives his penis as small when it is of normal size; he is reflecting in his body perception an introjected relationship with a father that played up the smallness or inferiority of his self and the consequent strength and superiority of the father. "Somehow," they say, "the penis becomes a focal representation for the characteristics of this system" (p. 353). This takes us in the direction of symptom—a topic I will consider later.

At the moment, I want to focus on the metaphoric outgrowths of bodily experience. A cornerstone article in this field was the work of a British psychoanalyst, Ella Sharpe (1968); her paper, "Psychophysical problems revealed in language: An examination of metaphor," originally published in 1940, has had to be taken into account by every psychoanalytic psychologist writing after her.

Sharpe starts by saying that "just as in the study of language we find that no word is metaphysical without its first having been physical, so our search when we listen to patients must be for the physical basis and experience from which metaphorical speech springs" (p. 156). Any live metaphor, she asserts, grows initially out of past psychophysical experiences, and metaphor originates when bodily experiences become controlled—especially those relating to bodily orifices. Emotions that originally went along with bodily discharge find alternative channels. Speech itself, she says, is a kind of metaphor: Words become the substitutes for the bodily discharge and can serve the function of a stream of urine, a smoke screen, gas, or "bleating."

In this early paper urging the fruitfulness of exploring metaphoric imagery, Sharpe (1968) writes:

When dynamic thought and emotional experiences of the for-
gotten past find the appropriate verbal image in the preconscious, language is as pre-determined as a slip of the tongue or
trick of behaviour. Metaphor, then, is personal and individual
even though the words and phrases used are not of the speaker's
coinage. (p. 159)

Thus, she holds that a metaphor spontaneously produced by a patient
may turn out to summarize an infantile experience, often, in her view,
reflecting pregenital and repressed oedipal wishes, and reflecting as
well something of the early environment that has been incorporated.

As examples of failed sucking experiences, she cites pervasive
references to losing something, not taking something in, and not
getting the point. Weaning, too, has its metaphors. A patient who in
being weaned was flung from her mother's breast to her bed, years later
takes as analogies for rifts in her adult relationships such violent
metaphors as being unhorsed, flinging or being flung aside, dropping.
Sharpe's general point is that these early experiences form the matrix
for adult perceptions of human relatedness, and they will often be
expressed in terms of the concrete physical sensations that initially
gave rise to them.

For example, when an infant has had a history of lying cold,
wet, and helpless in bed, this catastrophic psychophysical situation
will probably become the symbolic vehicle through which he later
describes depression. He may thus speak of feeling "sodden with
despair," being "in a rut of depression," or feeling "awash in troubles."

Going still further, Sharpe talks of bodily orifices taking on
metaphoric functions. The control of aggression symbolized by a taut
sphincter becomes a metaphor for control in general: "Unconscious
control of the bodily openings and the unconscious super-ego are then
inseparable. The super-ego takes on the quality of a physical sphincter, rigid, implacable, and merciless in judgment" (p. 165).

Although acknowledging the importance of Sharpe's contribution, I believe that she was too schematic and overgeneralizing. She
tends to give a too-simple drive-dominated interpretation in which
the metaphor is detached from a richer sense of the individual's
dynamic background and object relations. As a result, symbolic equations (in which x equals always and only y) come to dominate,
yielding standard meanings of metaphors for all patients. [This

reductionism recalls Ernest Jones's (1916) standard dictionary-like interpretations of dream symbols, which, in the name of science, actually restrict the power of metaphor.] Arlow (1979) in his important paper on metaphor takes Sharpe to task for this kind of reductionism.

Furthermore, it is unlikely that *all* metaphor arises in connection with early bodily experience. This view seems unnecessarily reductive of later experience that is not strictly somatically based. It seems plausible to me to suggest that *many*, rather than all, of the most charged metaphors we use originate from bodily experience, since the body is the ground of all our sensory life and hence through it we accumulate the raw material of our metaphor making.

IMAGES OF THE BODY CONTAINER IN RELATION TO PSYCHOSOMATIC SYMPTOMS

Through our bodies, we accumulate the raw material not only of metaphors but of their enactments (or em*bodi*ments) as psychosomatic symptoms. In an important study, Fisher and Cleveland (1968) hypothesized that the way in which individuals perceive their bodies would relate to the geography of their psychosomatic symptoms. Specifically, they predicted that patients with arthritis (which has been shown to have a large psychological loading) would focus on the edges and boundaries of percepts in the Rorschach. Conversely, those with psychosomatic gastrointestinal conditions would give responses not of barriers and boundaries but of things being entered or penetrated. These results were borne out, and a control study of patients with accidental, physical sources for similar symptoms did not show similar fixation on barriers or penetration. Thus, the causal arrow seems to show that a perceived defect in the body image leads to the psychosomatic symptom, and not the other way around.

We can see that psychological states are portrayed via body images. Sometimes they are portrayed as metaphors, as when depression is described as a sodden wetness; in that case, a mental state is being likened to the physical experience that gave rise to this state originally. In other cases, when symptoms arise from mental states, the body becomes the concrete manifestation or symbolic equivalent of the psychological condition.

SYMPTOM VERSUS METAPHOR

In his careful and lucid analysis of symptom and metaphor, Wright (1976) has written that "while *symptoms* reveal much about the *defensive* operations of the ego, and the kinds of structure that arise when the ego has 'refused' integration, *metaphor* reveals the ego in its creative operations and is a structure in whose formation the ego has fully participated" (p. 97). The presence or absence of ego integration parallels what we noted in contrasting dream images with metaphors. Both symptom and dream image reflect primary process in an unintegrated way, whereas metaphor typically integrates conscious and unconscious.

Basing his analysis primarily on phobic symptoms, Wright focuses on the formal structure rather than the content of metaphors and symptoms. He describes metaphor as a verbal structure that exists in a context of imagery, affect, and thought, while a symptom exists in a context of imagery, affect, and action. Thus, both share the components of image and affect, but metaphor is characterized by the inner experimental action of *thought*, whereas symptom is acted out through the body.

Wright (1976) tersely summarizes the distinctions between symptom and metaphor:

1. Both symbolic structures (metaphor and symptom) present one thing in the semblance of another; but whereas the symptom *conceals* and leads to a *restriction* of view, metaphor *reveals* and leads out to new vision.
2. The *symptom* is a wordless presentation of an unnameable dilemma—an abortive metaphor that stops below the level of speech.
3. *Metaphor* is a product of an ego that is going towards a problem and attempting to grasp it. *The symptom* is a product of an ego that is turning away from a problem and

refusing to see it. Whether symptom or metaphor arises depends on the *attitude of the ego* that is confronted with the problem.

4. The undoing of a symptom is in part the creation of *metaphor* from symptom.

Where id was there shall ego be.
Where symptom was there metaphor shall be. (p. 98)

"A symptom," writes Lacan (1977) "is a metaphor in which flesh or function is taken as the signifying element" (p. 166). This difference gets at what I feel to be the very heart of the process of depth psychotherapy: In a talking cure that uses words rather than enactments, the patient is urged to talk about rather than act out his or her psychological conflicts. Our patients are helped to work with and in a profound way to play with what besets them, rather than to embody it. They are helped to create metaphors out of symptoms.

TRANSFORMATION OF SYMPTOM INTO METAPHOR: A CASE EXAMPLE

To illustrate how a change of ego attitude can convert symptom into metaphor, I present the following case example, setting the symptom and its metaphoric evolution into the wider context of case history.

Martha D. is a woman I saw in therapy for seven years. She came to see me after hearing me give a talk on making major life changes in a workshop for people who had recently relocated. She was new to the Bay Area, having come from Chicago to be with her son, and leaving behind her a job, a circle of friends, some extended family, and a recently divorced husband. This was to be her venue for "starting over."

She called me for an initial appointment in panic when she realized that her son, a graduate student, was not about to take her in; she felt bereft and friendless and discontinuous from her midwestern life.

Martha is an extraordinarily articulate woman who had been schooled in how to talk by seven years of psychoanalysis, but the sense

I began to get was of her not quite being in the room with me. She had trouble looking at me, and for some time I could feel how intense her fear of engagement was by the way she needed to propitiate me—I was to be her savior who would miraculously deliver her, but all too often she experienced me as her judging mother; most of the time, I was someone to be held off with a volley of talk, so that I felt everything I said was an interruption. And she had to detoxify what I did say by telling me that she had already thought of that herself, or wasn't that funny, she had wondered that just the other day. She seemed to need to defend against invasion from me by feeling that whatever I said had originally come from inside herself.

Martha's father had been a diplomat stationed in Ceylon. Her mother went into a profound depression after the birth of Martha's two-year younger brother, Jamie. Martha remembers seeing the disheveled hair and distressed face of her mother when she returned from the hospital and not recognizing her. Indeed, she felt for a long time that she had lost her mother and that this hated little brother had taken away or malevolently changed her real mother. In the wake of the mother's deep depression, the family returned to Washington, D. C., where her father worked in the State Department and the family began trying to put the shards together. The mother did recover enough to function in a superficial way but spent much of her time withdrawing from the family, particularly the father, whom she regarded as a brute for forcing his sexual attentions on her.

Martha's relationship with her mother was extraordinarily close. She was the favored good child, whereas her brother was the bad, troublesome one. But this closeness was bought at the expense of an enormous sacrifice of Martha's real self. In ministering to her mother, coming into the bedroom to visit with her, she felt she had to follow a narrowly prescribed role: be cheerful and sympathetic, but not too boisterous; tone down whatever happened that was really good or exciting or disturbing; sympathize with mother's complaints about father; keep a low profile. Only outside the house could she laugh and play with friends along the banks of the Potomac. Inside, the house was like a mausoleum where she felt she must walk with her head bowed.

In the course of our work together, the splits that divided Martha's psyche became abundantly clear: She would either be saved or damned; I was either her rescuer or her condemning judge; she was either all bad and hence fit for the grossest punishment or had finally proved herself good enough to be redeemed. She talked about and then came to see how when people—especially men—failed to make her feel perfect and hence acceptable, she would, as she put it "X them out." Life seemed to be a desperate struggle between "X'ing out" and "being X'ed out." She told me poignantly how she had managed to fool people: being the competent, cheerful child protective services worker while inwardly feeling hollow. It was always a question of putting on a hat, of playing a role. She loathed being a caretaker, and yet she kept being driven back to that role. She did not work for the first five years of her therapy with me, drawing on the money she had received in her divorce settlement to live on.

Thus, for five years, she proceeded to spend virtually every cent of her savings, as she stayed at home, coming to see me regularly but otherwise living an almost monastic life that replicated her mother's long periods of retirement and seclusion. I felt a genuine panic at seeing her bankrupting herself, and it seemed to me that, as I told her, I was carrying the panic for her, while she appeared insouciantly to be going down the drain. It became clear to me from a brief period of unsatisfying work she had had a few years earlier that, distasteful as the social service work had been, it seemed to organize her and was, of course, necessary for her survival, and I talked with her about these feelings, knowing that I might well be perceived as "forcing" her to do work she hated.

At the point at which she would have had to go on welfare, this articulate, thoughtful, witty woman, with enormous unlived potential took a rather lowly job as a receptionist in a law office. This reemergence into the external world, underpinned by years of patient therapeutic work, seemed to be almost transformative.

For the first time, she was able to look at me as she talked and to allow me to say things she had not thought of first. For the first time, she was able to see her father in a more rounded way: not only as a bumbling loudmouth but as a man who had shown some tenderness to her and for whom she occasionally felt some tenderness as well. For the first time she could see an authority figure—her boss—as a whole person: neither devil nor demigod, but a good and flawed man: "He's really rather witty and a delight to talk to, but he has this awfully infantile side; knowing that makes me feel less like 'I'm all bad' when he yells at me and more like 'David's in one of his moods.' " This bit of assimilated reality and loss of omnipotence (if something bad happens to me it's because of my badness) may sound small enough, but Martha rightly experienced it as an enormous breakthrough. The miracle she had been yearning for in therapy was coming to pass. It was not salvation or redemption, it was the glimmerings of a new psychological world in which both the internal and the external could play a part: dreams and work-a-day reality, herself as a real person talking to me as a real person. A split two-dimensional world—like the two side-by-side pictures on a stereopticon slide—was becoming fused into a unified three-dimensional world with contours, depth, and roundness as her ego had become a more trustworthy instrument with which to view reality.

But healing these splits came at great cost, because what had caused the split in the first place seemed to be "clinging on" in an almost personified way. It was connected somehow with her mother and her mother's split view of the world, and it took a bodily form that seemed a most eloquent and concrete metaphor for what was happening in Martha's psyche: a clamping down in her midsection. This would occur whenever she began putting together what had been kept apart and particularly when seeing herself or me in a more complex, differentiated, *and* unified way, or whenever she felt more complex affects toward her parents than she had ever admitted: contempt for her mother as well as concern, tenderness for her father as well as scorn, compassion for her brother as well as rage. Whenever this happened, her body would attempt to say "No, thou shalt not connect." The symptom took the form of experiencing a tight rubber band around her midsection, which seemed at those moments to be clamped taut all around so that her body felt almost literally disconnected, top from bottom, head from viscera. This clamp of tension would then effectively sever the connection she had just made. It could happen when she began connecting affects with ideas, that is, really feeling her experiences as she had not been able to do for the years in which she simply intellectualized about them. When that kind of connection did occur, followed by the experiencing of the band, she would almost always say, "And now it's time to leave."

At that point we were able to explore the sensation and its implications first at the most real and literal level—the cutting off of her viscera from her ceaselessly working brain. In addition, I could help her consider the symbolic aspects, and the body metaphor gave us the clue and the opportunity to talk about it while it was happening in the room.

Martha began to see that she could either perceive her mother as lovingly merged or as hostilely opposed but not as someone embodying both the good and terrifying maternal aspects. Similarly, she could see me as the good mother only when she could shut off my physical presence. She described feeling really connected to me when she was at home and would have long imaginary conversations with me; then I could be experienced in my benign aspect: as audience, guide, and loving caregiver. But in the room, as I have said, for years she experienced me very differently: I was the negative mother who might criticize, attack, and belittle her. What struck me in all this was her loyalty to her dead mother as though looking at me and realizing I was *not* her mother would have been a kind of heresy and betrayal to her internalized mother. On the other hand, if I *were* her mother I would somehow attack her or my gaze would turn her to stone. And indeed, this band inside her sometimes felt like taut rubber, but more often felt like concrete—a stone partition that cut her in two.

What this metaphor served to highlight for both of us was how painfully dangerous it was to connect and how strong was the pull to disconnect. In a late hour she said, "I just realized I was expecting my boss to attack me, and I see that by being so suspicious, I may in fact, be inviting some attack." Such a differentiated statement, which involved the assumption of appropriate but not omnipotent responsibility, would have been unthinkable much earlier. Yet even then when Martha actually became aware of what she had just said, she experienced the bodily metaphor: "Clamp. Disconnect. I'm doing it again." Or another time: "My whole midsection is going like this" (she holds up a clenched fist). "Like it's saying, 'Don't see, don't see.' " And again:

Connecting is what I have to do, and if my body is refusing, it's just my body. I hear a voice say, "At 59, why bother?" It's the voice of my inner saboteur. And I answer, "Because I have nothing to do in my life that's better or more important."

This she said with tears in her eyes and a voice fierce in its determination.

So the forces for connecting had become stronger, and the split *was* healing. The band—rubber or concrete—was not so acutely felt, and it relaxed its hold sooner. And at least once, the meaning of the band was glossed by an image that followed in its wake spontaneously. No sooner had Martha "disconnected" than she saw a sudden vivid image: her mother with wings swooping down on her and suffocating her. "Wings are usually associated with angels, but in this case, it—she—was a devil. And of course, Lucifer himself was a fallen angel. It was my mother after Jamie was born." This dramatically illustrated the split in her perception of her mother (angel or devil) and the impact of the change caused by the mother's psychotic depression after her brother was born: a discontinuity that became the basic paradigm of herself and the world.

I was able to help her see how the symptom of the band was using the body to represent a psychological state, that is, how much a metaphor it could become. She came to see the dangers the band was aimed to forestall: To connect the good and the bad destroys the good; to connect to the outer world could rob her of her inner world; to see me as a whole person threatened to overwhelm the good in me with the bad and to break the symbiotic tie with her mother.

By the end of the treatment, the band was only a momentary twinge. It was a cue that indicated Martha was about to disconnect; but it was now a signal that her ego could register and override. This somatic equivalent of splitting became a focal and viable metaphor that proved central in our therapeutic work together.

INSIGHT AS CONNECTION THROUGH BODY AFFECT

In a famous passage in E. M. Forster's *Howard's End* (1921), the heroine says,

> Only connect! That was the whole of her sermon. Only con-
> nect the prose and the passion, and both will be exalted . . .
> Live in fragments no longer. Only connect, and the beast and
> the monk, robbed of the isolation that is life to either, will die.
> (p. 187)

This seems to be a way of saying, "Where id and superego were [the beast, the monk], there shall ego be." And furthermore, what better way to describe cognition and affect respectively than "the prose and the passion"?

Psychoanalyst Leonard Shengold (1981) maintains that it is this vital connection of prose and passion that constitutes insight. Neither alone will do it: Cognition without affect is simply an intellectualization that will not hold; affect without cognition is just a feeling-state without a home.

Shengold, in examining insight as metaphor and the metaphor that embodies insight, emphasizes the primary importance of body experience in these connections. He illustrates with a case of his own. The patient, who was provocative and isolated and felt more comfortable with his angry than his loving feelings, continually kept the analyst at bay. Yet Shengold knew that despite the patient's distancing maneuvers and his allowing closeness only in the form of wrestling matches, the patient valued the analytic experience intensely.

Shengold (1981) describes a session in which the patient for the first time calmly said that he realized his analyst was a good, kind person but one he hated nonetheless. This, the author notes, was the beginning of an emotional change: The "good" feeling that makes the patient feel unprotected can at last be spoken, even though only the hatred is truly known. The patient then spoke of a fantasied triangle at work, and about how his talk about triangles had always had an abstract, intellectual quality:

> But today, somehow I feel that triangle and how it relates to my father and mother; I feel it in three dimensions. [This is said with excitement and involvement.] I feel the good feelings, and the bad feelings; the sex, and the jealousy. It's all mixed up, but it's real. It's not bad or good, it's bad-and-good. I hate my father, and I love my father. You know this sounds like fancy intellectual stuff, but today it is different. It is all real and palpable; it's like a bowel movement. (p. 300)

This fecal metaphor was experienced by the patient, close to tears, as an "epiphany." The analyst noted to himself the regressive associations, the wrestling matches of the present antedated by wrestling over bowel training; and in the archaic past of the patient, the bowel movement was simultaneously me/not-me, inside/outside. These were themes for later exploration.

But in the session in question, the patient showed that he had made connections intellectually while still being able to grasp the "palpableness" of psychological reality: "Primary process was felicitously intertwined with secondary process. The 'anal grasp' of the bowel movement by his anal sphincter which had emerged from the unconscious to supply an experiential component of memory was facilitating the grasp of the ego" (p. 300). This overwhelming experience of wholeness occurred as the patient experienced himself *and* his father *and* his analyst in a simultaneously more differentiated and more integrated way.

The important point is that although the hour was the result of many previous hours of working through, it seemed to pivot on the metaphor of the bowel movement as "the real and palpable." With this breakthrough of what could be called body affect into the defensive barrier or wrapping, the patient found himself in a different place. This place Shengold describes metaphorically as a "labyrinth of metaphor." (The bodily base for *Shengold's* choice of the labyrinth metaphor may have been an association to the intestinal labyrinth which the patient's metaphor touched off in him.) The patient's metaphor, with its insistent bodily physicality, brought with it an enormous sense of conviction and affective rightness.

At the end of Chapter 1, I noted the connection between metaphor and affect. Now we can push the connection a step further: One reason that metaphors flow from and evoke affect is because they originate mainly from our most primary experiences of and with our own bodies. This bodily experience determines our image of the world around us.

The primary metaphorical connections between the body ego and the external world—links whose initial forging were so fraught with affect and with vivid sensation—are, according to Shengold (1981), "the first steps toward our thought, language, memory and insight. Metaphor in this sense marks the beginning and continuing road of the journey of our life" (p. 302). It takes us back to the time of what Mahler et al. (1975) call "the psychological birth of the human infant," the time when inside and outside, body and external world, self and objects (especially parents) are first differentiated and then connected. These connections, when accompanied by the fervid affect they originally had can truly be called insights.

Shengold reminds us of Freud's dictum that exploratory work is not directed squarely at the unconscious or experiential origins but "at some place above 'the roots of the phenomena . . . at a point which has been made *accessible* to us . . .' " (p. 304). Metaphor provides close-in presently available experience that becomes a transitional phenomenon linking one's inner (originally bodily) experience and the outer world.

Our circuit through the bodily base of metaphor and its grounding in the body image has, I hope, shown how the basic functional operation of metaphor—connection—is a crucial dimension of both physical and psychological life. It is also the paradigmatic experience of the work of therapy: True insight is always connection, a simultaneous experience of feeling and thought, of "passion and prose." How patients can be helped to connect with even seemingly casual or trivial metaphors will form the substance of the next chapter in a close look at the process of particularly fruitful hours.

CHAPTER 3

Exploring the Sources of Metaphors Clinically

> . . . metaphor can regularly be seen as an outcropping of unconscious fantasy. Specific associations to the metaphor regularly lead to an unconscious fantasy typical for the patient . . . [T]his held true whether the metaphor was vitally innovative and expressive or of a stale, cliché quality.
>
> —JACOB ARLOW, "Metaphor and the Psychoanalytic Situation"

CONVENTIONAL OR AUTOMATIC METAPHORS

How much of the time we sit in our offices and listen to our patients use what seem to be the clichés of psychological experience! They talk of feeling trapped, of having a wall go up, of being fenced in or of being suffocated. They talk of a breakthrough. In listening, we often do not see the metaphor but look through it or past it, to the content it appears to address. These clichés may have been born originally out of bodily experience that was once vivid and compelling. But now the figures appear worn out—like coins so thumbed one can scarcely distinguish the buffalo's head on the old nickel.

Yet many of these wornout metaphors are unconsciously determined figurative expressions that may have a vivid sensory connection and the potential for affective charge. Furthermore, although the unconscious fantasy to which the metaphor is linked may not be fully retrievable, we can certainly learn more about the unconscious source and dynamics of the metaphor.

Before discussing these conventional metaphors—ones that are tossed off lightly and without deliberation—I would like to introduce a distinction made by Kenneth Wright (1976). He calls the vivid metaphor that retains its contact with an affect-laden image an "integrated" metaphor. Such metaphors, I have found, announce themselves in dramatic, deliberate ways: They take center stage and demand attention. An example would be the butterfly metaphor I cited in Chapter 1, and I will mention others when I talk about "key" metaphors and "metaphors of the self." These figures are clearly connected to their train of image and affect, both of which are very close to consciousness.

Next there is what Wright calls the "pale metaphor," which arouses some imagery but seems at first glance to be cut off from affect. These are often embedded metaphors: They do not herald themselves directly. In fact, they are tossed off in passing almost casually. Nevertheless, they often point to a personal image that can yield its affect upon exploration (see the "ghost" metaphor below).

At the point of lowest psychological energy is what Wright calls a "faded" (and I call a "conventional") metaphor. Here even the imagery seems to have died off, and the metaphor looks like pure cliché—phrases such as "I am blocked," or "He was picking on me." (I am reminded that the term "cliché" itself is actually a metaphor: Originally it referred, in French, to the stereotype plate used in printing to reproduce page after page without variation.)

I certainly would not explore every such conventional metaphor (and I will cite in Chapter 7 the case of what seems to me to be a too-zealous pursuit of metaphor). But I do keep my ears open for derivatives and possibilities for reviving both the image and the affect that are sleeping within the walls and fences our patients surround themselves with. It takes therapeutic skill to know when to climb the wall or to enter the prison in imagination and when to wait until these metaphoric images arise more persistently or dynamically. Often subtle affective cues from the patient will provide guidance. Of course, the best guide is one's thorough knowledge of the patient so that we can notice changes from their baselines in expression, tone of voice, emphasis, or body language, or anything that is novel in the interpersonal field when a metaphor is introduced.

ENLIVENING THE
CONVENTIONAL METAPHOR

I have found that even metaphors that appear to be entirely automatic are often merely slumbering and that they can be awakened and made to yield up their living connections with image, fantasy, and memory. Which of these metaphors to explore is a question that has to do with the artful aspect of psychotherapy, requiring tact, a knowledge of this particular patient, and an informed intuition about where to look for gold among the rocks.

I want to give two examples of seemingly innocuous metaphors that could easily have gone unnoticed but that in both cases led to important material that otherwise might not have come up so directly or with so much affect. In fact, I believe that once one's metaphoric sensitivity has been honed, any metaphor *can* serve to open these wider or deeper vistas. As W. H. Auden put it, "The crack in the teacup opens/ A lane to the land of the dead." Auden's metaphor bears looking at for what it tells us about the symbolic process. In the poem from which these lines come, "As I Walked Out One Evening," Auden talks about two lovers, entwined in one another's arms, and oblivious to the eroding work of time; but another world of phantasms and incongruities lies below the lovers' apparent world (much as the unconscious with all its strange reversals, contradictions, anomalies underlies the conscious rational one). The slightest hint can often open up huge—and sometimes frightening—vistas. This is, in fact, what happened with each of the two patients I will describe.

Case Example: "He Was Picking on Me"

A 25-year-old woman, a landscape architect I will call Brigitte D., is a volatile redhead in her mid-20s with a slight accent reflecting her French Canadian birthplace. She has told me about her sudden rages and her fear of men. In one session, she found herself getting violently angry at her boyfriend's jealousy, which she was somewhat consciously evoking. She tells me about a fight they had had the previous day. He began interrogating her about another man, and she ended by hitting him. Then she got terrified of her own behavior and fled the scene.

"I felt, you know, that he was right in a way to accuse me of hiding things from him and of not telling this other guy about my commitment to him, but I also felt he was—how you say, *picking* on me."

She seemed to italicize the word as she spoke. In other circumstances, I might have let the conventional metaphor go, but she gave me a *gestural cue* that something affectively important was happening: She illustrated the metaphor bodily by gouging her left arm with the fingers of her right hand. Acting on that cue, I simply underlined the metaphor by reiterating it as a question: "Picking on you?"

"Yes," she said. "Examining me with picks."

I immediately knew from both her physical gesture and the vividness of the image that this was no automatic metaphor, as when we say unthinkingly, "Quit picking on me." So I asked her to tell me what that feeling was like, and what if anything she had been seeing as she had told me that.

"Well, I actually had an image of him, you know, dissecting me."

I knew from Brigitte's history that this intense image was based on a sense of being helpless and alternately worshipped and sadistically treated in her family. I also wondered if anything in the transference was giving rise to those feelings. Had *I* been picking on her? I could not find any warrant in our relationship at the moment to pursue that notion. So I asked her to tell me more about "dissecting."

"Like I was stretched out on a table and he was, I don't know, probing, cutting me open, cutting me all over." She shuddered and covered her face with her hands, and I waited for her feelings to subside.

"It sounds as though you felt you were in the hands of a mad surgeon," I said.

She nodded vigorously. "Yes, that *is* what it felt like. And just now I am realizing that that's of course precisely how I felt with my father. That's exactly, you know, how *he* would grill me when I was a teenager, you know, *pick* at me. Where had I been? Who had I been out with? What had we done?"

I said, continuing with the metaphor, "And you would feel paralyzed. Like an anesthetized patient."

"Well, yes, I *felt* paralyzed. But then I'd have to try to do something—anything. Sometimes I'd just run away. Sometimes I would try to fight back. But with my father, you could never win."

I understood that her only alternative to being paralyzed, then as now, was flight or fight.

Brigitte then talked about her adolescent experience of her father: his excessive curiosity and possessiveness of her, his unreasonableness, and his inability to negotiate. Not only were his rules arbitrary, but they seemed to be always changing: one month her curfew would be at 11:00 P.M. on weekends with no going out during the week; the next month, she would only be allowed out one night of the weekend, and so on.

It became clear that in all her dealings with men, their perceived sexual curiosity and intrusiveness were highly salient for her. The larger implications of this sense of being sadistically invaded and operated on surfaced some weeks later when I was exploring the meaning of a check she had given me that had bounced. As we talked both about her actual financial situation and the symbolic implications of the bounced check, it was clear that she was seeing me in a similar way, as cutting her open and grilling her. She was able to see at that point how I too had begun to seem like a mad surgeon and that that indeed was a metaphoric template she often applied—usually to men, but also to women when she felt threatened by them.

As our work progressed, she began to differentiate when the metaphor was being used appropriately and when it was not, or, more accurately, to differentiate her inner experience of being dissected from the intent of the other person. This was particularly difficult because, shortly after the session I have described, she remembered something she had repressed for years—that a farmhand had repeatedly sexually molested her when she was 11 and threatened her if she told her family. So she had indeed been invaded and picked apart.

The rest of the therapy consisted partly of attempts to help her work through that trauma and to see how her present behavior at times could provoke the very attacking response she so feared but that felt so familiar from the time when she had been, indeed, a passive victim and when the probing or invasion had truly been beyond her control.

This material might have come up in other ways, but it had not. Brigitte was a highly outer-directed person who had never reported a dream or a fantasy directly. With such patients, metaphor is also characteristically conventional. Nevertheless, to the attentive listener even such a "dead" metaphor can be an important conduit to material that has been buried alive and inaccessible through other routes. Its exploration requires a temporary immersion in the patient's experience of the figure, a taking of it "as if" it were real.

Case Example: "I Feel Ghostly"

Another metaphoric image that opened a lane to the land of memory and feeling was provided by a highly articulate woman I will call Margaret E., a fair, petite writer in her late 40s. I had seen Margaret for about a year, and during this particular session she had been talking uninterruptedly for some time as I sat quietly listening.

She was telling me how hard it has been for her to acknowledge her own power. "It's hard in the outside world, hard with Tim [her husband], and sometimes hard with you too. I have moments of feeling impotent and unreal. At times, like right now, I feel ghostly."

She began to pursue another topic, but I knew Margaret's style by then. I knew that, unlike Brigitte, she tended to use figurative language with great precision. So when she spoke of herself as "ghostly," I intuited that she was trying to tell me something important and new. Upon that cue, I said:

"That's the first time I've heard you describe yourself that way—as ghostly. It must be a very uncomfortable feeling."

She told me it *was* upsetting to feel ghostly, and I asked her, as I often do in exploring a metaphor, if she had an image in mind when she was telling me that.

"Oh, I don't know—pale, amorphous, even unreal. . . . I guess I'd have to say without boundaries, hazy and white. It makes me think of a dream that recurred almost nightly when I was four or five. I dreamt of bodies, a whole host of bodies, all bound in strips of cloths, in bandages, like the mummies I'd seen at the Museum of Natural History. They weren't just lying there, as the Egyptian mummies had lain in their sarcophagi. No, these were walking-around mummies. But silent. I couldn't see any faces.

"I would have this dream, I seem to remember, almost every night. And when I awoke, I was so terrified, my heart jolted, and I'd grab for Tidsy, my precious teddy bear. I guess this dream recurred—but less frequently—even through high school. It began around four—the year I had my tonsils out.

"Come to think of it, the dream must have started right after that. My mother later told me she had been afraid of upsetting me if she told me much about the operation in advance. So what she did—well, she—actually, she tricked me into going to the hospital. She told me later she did it so I wouldn't be upset far in advance. But I think she couldn't deal with my being anxious for any length of time. She was terrified of strong feelings—hers, mine, or anyone's. That's part of why she drank. Anyhow, what she told me was that I would be her assistant and work in the hospital library where she did volunteer work. I remember dimly her telling me this, and I know I was excited. But then suddenly they were putting a white hospital robe on me and wheeling me away from her. A door swung shut, and I was in a room with what seemed to me a bunch of ghosts. They must have been wearing hospital greens, the nurses and doctors, but my memory is of a bunch of shrouded masked figures all in white. As the sickly sweet cone came down over my face—was it ether they used then?—I kicked and screamed in panic. The anesthesiologist told my mother he had never seen a child fight an anesthetic so. Or so she told me."

"No wonder," I said. "After that horrendous deception by your mother, you were wheeled away from her and suddenly surrounded by those ghostly presences. You would have felt absolute terror—the terror of not-being."

"Oh, *yes!*" she said. "It was worse than the worst nightmare." She paused for awhile, lost in her memories, then resumed. "You know that dream about the mummies continued almost all the way through high school? And even to this day I have to sleep with a light on. Tim teases me about it, but I can't sleep in the dark. I don't know what I'm afraid of—arsonists? burglars?"

"Or ghosts?" I asked, returning to the original metaphor. (I felt the material here had something to do with her mother who may indeed have been experienced more as a vampire than an ordinary ghost, but I wanted to wait till she was closer to her feelings about this to interpret it. So I merely harked back to the original metaphor.)

"Ghosts are actually more terrifying to me in dreams than a real person coming at me violently. More menacing. In my dreams, the ghosts seem to be both there and not there," she said.

She shivered and then told me she was suddenly remembering going when she was very little to the funeral of her very old great-aunt Margaret whose namesake she was. Her great-aunt was lying in an open coffin, and her father urged Margaret to kiss her great-aunt's cheek. She could feel even now, she told me, the unearthly coldness of that dead cheek. And she still had the fear that if someone—a dog, her teenage daughter, her husband—is very quiet, she has to check and make sure they are not dead.

"As you did with your mother," I said, remembering what she had told me about her mother's stupors.

"You know, I've tried to forget that stuff. Not to remember or face up to her drinking or the depression that led to it. I know that when my father was out on the road selling for weeks at a time, she'd come into my bed at night completely plastered. She'd be so out of it that when she slept, it was like a coma, and there was no way I could rouse her. I would call her and sometimes shake her, and she still didn't wake up. She was a zombie. And I was so scared: I wouldn't know if she was dead or alive." She began to cry.

I felt for what Margaret must have experienced as a terrified child, desperately needing reassurance and knowing that the one person who could possibly comfort her was either completely unavailable or possibly, worse still, dead. I believe my face and my body conveyed this empathic understanding to her without words. She sat crying for awhile and then said, somewhat bitterly, "A ghost among ghosts. . . . that's what I feel like sometimes."

A bit later, after she had recovered, I said, "I'm remembering that at the point in the hour when you first brought up feeling ghostly, I had been very quiet. Perhaps you were wondering if I, too, was a ghost who was and was not here at the same time."

She smiled at that point, and I knew my intervention had connected. "Well, yes, I think that idea was flickering around the edge of my consciousness. In fact, maybe that's what started it. At times you do seem to recede and I have trouble knowing if you're really there." (This was the most "critical" thing she had been able to bring herself to say to me in our year of working together.)

"But I have to say," she grinned, "most of the time you seem pretty darn solid."

I acknowledged that that was indeed important, but that we also had to recognize her still-hovering fear of my impermanence. And, in fact, I was able to use my heightened sensitivity on this score in the further unfolding of the therapy to track her experience of me, particularly during my silences or impending vacations, as the ghostly mother. In the course of that work, I was led to recall the perceptive dictum of Loewald (1960) that in the work of analysis, "ghosts are transformed into ancestors" (p.29).

UNEARTHING THE ROOTS OF A CONVENTIONAL METAPHOR

The following is an example in which the unconscious of the patient triggered images in the therapist that became the ground for understanding and interpreting. The hour could be seen as variations on a submerged theme.

Case Example: "I Feel Totally Unequipped"

My patient, Dodie R., was a strikingly tall, slim woman in her mid-30s who had recently married a somewhat older very successful lawyer and was working at her first job after getting a master's degree in vocational rehabilitation. This was a huge step for her because, although she is very quick, she comes from a working-class milieu in which no one went beyond high school, and, indeed, successful people were often disparaged. People who made it were accused by her father's family of "having pull" or doing something "crooked."

Dodie, after an abortive marriage in her 20s and several relationships that followed a sacrificial pattern, had found a man who is strong and stable, unlike the men in her family of origin. She felt for the first time that the underpinnings of her everyday life were secure enough to enable her to look at her persistent free-floating anxiety and her blocks about taking risks or asserting herself.

In the course of our first months of working together, Dodie did some remarkable and difficult things. She confronted her mother about her depressive episodes not in anger but in sorrow, with the result that her mother agreed to seek professional help. She also began piecing together the circumstances of her early life by pressing her mother for information. Exploring the mist that had surrounded her early years, she found out that her father had been in the service in Korea when she was little and that her mother had raised her alone and had had a prolonged depressive episode. She showed me a picture of herself at two, a beautiful but forlorn child being held stiffly by her gaunt mother.

In looking for men who would redeem her or whom she could redeem, she has in some sense also been looking for a way to release the energetic and "masculine" aspects of herself, so hidden under her facade of the beautiful, somewhat helpless woman.

In a session nearly a year into the therapy, Dodie began by talking about her discomfort about a comment made to her by the chairman of a mental health association on whose board she serves. At the end of a meeting the day before, during which she had made what she thought was a very inadequate presentation of local mental health funding needs, the chairman of the board told her, "You'll be sitting in this chair some day." She said that far from gratifying or assuring her, his statement plunged her into panic and made her want to flee.

I was proceeding at the time on the assumption that a grandiose fantasy had been triggered off and scared her, that the thought of outdistancing her depressed mother was too terrifying to contemplate, and that she had quickly cut her sails and experienced only helplessness. This may indeed have been the case, but in following the process of the hour, I heard other themes emerging, themes that called out to be honored and explored rather than fitted into the template in my head.

Dodie continued by saying how hard she found it to believe she could do anything really well. She produced a series of memories of her father's denigration of her competence. She remembered trying to do her arithmetic homework in grammar school. He was trying to help her with fractions but was pretty rusty himself. At one point, he got so exasperated he hit her over the head with the math book. She then recalled that when he had played catch with her and her younger brother, every time she threw the ball underhand, he would bark at her, "Can't you do *anything* right?"

"Maybe there were times," she told me, "when he wasn't like that, though I can't remember his *ever* encouraging me. I don't know if he really hated me or was just mad at the moment, but, honest, I heard such contempt and hatred in his voice."

I said, to underscore the inner effect of these experiences, that it was almost as though she was being *prohibited* from succeeding at anything.

"Well, yeah—" she said, "except maybe for being pretty and quiet. I did all my crying in my room by myself; I'd never be caught dead crying in front of them. That's why it's so hard for me to cry in front of you, even. And I guess that's why I have such trouble taking risks: I feel totally unequipped."

The word "unequipped" is a bland word, a cliché about incapacity. But without being fully conscious of the process, I must have made some association to phallic woundedness because the simile I then intuitively offered her carried connotations of castration expressed as bodily deformity. I said, "It's like a person with one short leg competing in an Olympic track race." And, indeed, she had been wounded in the domain of achievement and competitive striving.

Just as, in T. S. Eliot's view, "genuine poetry can communicate before it is understood," so metaphors, speaking from the unconscious of the patient to the unconscious of the therapist and vice versa, can communicate before they are fully understood. I, for example, did not spell out the phallic thrust of her embedded metaphor or of my simile, but Dodie showed me by the associations that followed that she had "heard" our interchange at a preconscious or unconscious level. Thus, not everything needs to be interpreted directly; often (as I will show in Chapter 5) we can sustain the therapeutic dialogue by staying "within the metaphor."

"Yes," said Dodie, "my father called me a total loss. I never thought about that before. Total loss. . . . Hmmmm. . . . That means he had no hope for me, and I had no hope either." She paused and began to cry quietly—the first time she had allowed herself to do so in my presence. After a bit she said, "It was like all I could do was just—just lie on the floor." Her brown eyes were still awash with tears.

We sat with our mutual images of her, as a child, on the floor. And at what seemed the right moment, I said, "As though you were a basket case."

"Oh, *yes!*" Dodie assented.

And suddenly she brightened, both because she felt understood and because something had suddenly become clear to her, both in her head and in her heart:

"You know, I *am* handicapped. It's true. It's a mental handicap, and that makes it harder to see than a physical handicap, but it's just as powerful. No, more powerful, because people don't watch out for you or make way for you the way they do for somebody who's got a physical handicap. But I know that for me to take even a small risk—well, it feels like an enormous thing. And I don't know if it will ever change."

I observed that she still feels often like a lost cause, a basket case.

She then recalled a dream she had had two nights earlier in which she had been watching a parade of retarded children—some lame and some cerebral palsied walking jaggedly through a small town. And in the dream, she found that she was not just observing but was walking with them; she was one of them.

We spent some time contemplating this dream, attending to the feelings it had evoked. I have found in my experience as an analysand as well as in my own clinical work that metaphors of wounded or deformed children are especially potent vehicles for affect and that each of us carries an image of his or her wounded inner child.

This wounded child image or theme was in the air from the moment Dodie entered the office that day, and both of us were resonating to it from the beginning to the end of the hour. The hour had a particular flavor—painful, tearful. It was like a musical "key" that was supplied by the incidental metaphor of being unequipped, which then modulated to the much more minor (and prevailing) key of being psychologically wounded. That key, supplied by that metaphor, calls for certain kinds of resonant responses: a cognitive intervention during that particular hour would have felt extremely jarring.

But at other times, when the "wounded child/basket case" theme was not so dominant or fraught, I could approach this metaphor in a different way. So, for example, I was aware of how Dodie wounds and disparages herself by "playing dumb," colluding with her father's view of her as she perceived it when young. I helped her see how her repeated "I don't knows" (she would typically begin a statement about herself with "I don't know why it is but . . .") were a product of her compliance with this ineffectual image of herself, and a way of not thinking for herself while submitting to me as the (father-) therapist. After some time, she became much more aware of this defensive stance, and could therefore label it herself and eventually subvert or circumvent it: "I'm saying 'I don't know,' and in a minute, I'll probably tell you just what's going on with me." This, said with a grin, was a first recognition of her considerable power to think and to understand.

I also knew that with this kind of wounding, eventually we would get to the plant onto which the father's disparagement was grafted and "took"—namely, the experience of herself as wounded through a mother who was isolated and depressed during most of Dodie's infancy.

These metaphors cast their shadows backward to childhood and forward to the working through in therapy. But what I want to emphasize here is a more microscopic view: that within an hour, a metaphor can create a kind of vibrational field—a force-field that attracts disparate particles and arranges them in lines of force around a magnetic core. To change the metaphor, after I, responding to "totally unequipped," introduced the image of physical handicap, this image became the leitmotif of the rest of the session. It became a leitmotif without any forcing or conscious willing on my part or presumably on hers, as a note that is sounded in one instrument may be picked up by "sympathetic vibrations" in a neighboring instrument. The therapist can receive the core image by an attitude of openness and, indeed, by *not* forcing but rather by allowing.

A NOVEL METAPHOR BECOMES A KEY METAPHOR

I want to give an example here of a metaphor that although not conventional or automatic like the ones mentioned previously did not reveal at first how crucial it was to the patient's concept of his entire self. I have called these "key metaphors," and will have more to say in the next chapter about how such metaphors of the self change in the course of therapy.

Case Example: "My Life Is a Pie"

A consultee presented the following material to me, as part of an ongoing consultation, and I include it here with his permission because it exemplifies how a sensitivity to exploring metaphor can result in the evocation of deep affect and focal issues. (I have taken the precaution here as elsewhere of disguising details that would identify the patient.)

The patient, whom I will call Michael C., was described to me as a tall balding unmarried 38-year-old advertising account executive. He had been more or less depressed for most of his life, but his depression increased after the death of his alcoholic father four years before he entered therapy. Michael's birth had coincided with the onset of angina in his mother, leaving the mother very little physical energy for the new baby.

For years, Michael has lived out a "false-self" accommodation— being nice, obliging, shaping himself to the needs of other people, including the psychologically disabled women with whom he has had brief relationships. The patient is, in Jungian typological terms, a feeling, intuitive type, who was born into an academic family in which thinking and rationality were the only currency acceptable. Judgments based on feeling simply "got in the way" and had to be expunged. So he was forced to deny his essential nature in an attempt to gain love and respect. In fact, several years into the course of the therapy he said, in what my consultee described as a stark and awful realization, "If I am myself, I kill my parents."

For years, the therapy went slowly, ploddingly, the patient's relationship to the therapist largely unspoken about, and transference interpretations so defended against that I recommended backing off until Michael was ready to experience more consciously both his attachment and his negative feelings toward my consultee. Michael did say that the therapist's office was the only place he did not have to try to be cheerful, accommodating, and nice. Still, he never seemed to ask for anything more than attention and an occasional reflective comment. The therapist often felt useless and helpless amidst the patient's generalized woe. I tried to help him understand how informative his countertransference was: He was feeling what the patient himself felt now and earlier. I indicated how important it was that for a time—perhaps a long time—he simply witness and allow Michael's despair without attempts to rescue or reason him out of it.

A highly intelligent man who *can* think symbolically, Michael described dreams and feeling states in which he seemed to be in a tunnel, walled off from a full life in one of the imprisoning but safe places we often hear about.

Aside from the tunnel, which actually arose from a dream image, Michael did not typically use figurative language in his therapeutic sessions. By the third year of treatment, the therapist was noting some changes, some increase in autonomy; one of his more cognitive interventions had helped the patient realize that it was not the first level of his depressing thoughts that was bothersome, it was what he came to call "the extras"—the catastrophizing extensions— that could plunge him into despair for days. Thus, it was not thinking "I feel lonely tonight" that was so hard to bear, it was the over-generalizing from this that Beck (1967) and others have pointed out that troubled him ("And therefore I'll never attract a woman again. And I'll be alone for the rest of my life. . . .")

By means of constant vigilance and by learning to talk to himself in a less self-defeating way, Michael was able to contain the scope of his despair, but I continued to share with the consultee my belief that the core problems of his depression had not been touched. He would stoutly insist that although he was having these difficulties that made him feel perpetually estranged from himself and that caused him either to grit his teeth while smiling or, when taxed past the point of smiling, to erupt angrily at coworkers, he was basically okay.

Through the therapeutic work, through slowly growing confidence in the therapist and the trust that he could receive steady, benign caring from him, Michael began to take a few risks: One of them was to attend a meeting of Adult Children of Alcoholics. At first his attitude was that of skeptical observer: His family had been upper-middle class and less disheveled on the surface than most of the families he heard about in ACA. It was as though he was simply being a tourist. But as he got the courage to speak and could really take in what the others were saying, he realized that, indeed, he was one of them, and that the denied and disguised alcoholism of his father ("He never fell down, he rarely missed his classes, he never physically abused us") had made things even more difficult and ambiguous for him.

The deepening of the therapeutic work itself was heralded by the patient's explicit use of a metaphor for himself—the first time this had happened in therapy. He had talked of feeling as if he were in a tunnel, but his insisting on the as-ifness of that metaphor distanced him from the emotional experience. In the session I will describe, however, he introduced a metaphor for his entire psyche. This is rather like the difference between saying "I'm in a tunnel" and "I *am* a tunnel." Metaphors that represent a symbolic equivalent to the self are particularly potent harbingers of psychological depth.

I will reconstruct from my consultation notes the part of the session in which the metaphor appeared in order to show how it became the nodal point of the hour and of how it represented, in Arlow's (1979) words, "an outcropping of unconscious fantasy" (p. 370).

Michael came in talking about having gone to Weight Watchers because he is somewhat overweight but not, according to my consultant, as much so as he feels himself to be. He says he used to play squash with some men at work, but he never seems to find time now, and he's feeling flabby as well as fat. At the Weight Watchers group meeting he felt uncomfortable at being one of the few men there and relieved that his weight problem was pretty slight compared to most of the others. But when they suggested that everyone present needed to try to give up sugar for life, he blanched. "That was just too stringent. Besides, that much of an addict I'm not. It's only when I'm depressed or restless that I OD on sweets."

This overture sounded the theme of oral deprivation that the therapist recognized; he hoped it would lead to similar and deeper material. And indeed, a metaphor combining sweets and devouring appeared in Michael's next association:

"I've often thought of my life as a pie," he said. "A whole, round pie, with only one piece missing." This association came as a surprise to the therapist, and he felt it was flagging something important since this man had rarely used explicit metaphors before. It should be noted that the first such deliberate use of a novel metaphor in a patient who rarely uses metaphor at all typically signals the emergence of highly charged material. The therapist wondered to himself what Michael would do with this figure.

"The one missing piece was a relationship—or at least, that's how my mother would have seen it. Now, I'm beginning to see it differently: Now I think it's not just one slice. Something has eaten a hole through the center of the pie, so that *each piece* is affected by it."

As he talked about this recognition of damage, Michael became choked up and lowered his head. After a bit he said tentatively, "I want your help and your advice." This was the first direct request he had ever made for psychological feeding by the therapist. But asking for the help rather than being heroically in charge was hard for him, so in the material that followed, the therapist had trouble finding out what kind of help Michael actually wanted. The patient talked about knowing that he should not wish to be taken care of but should try to learn how to take care of himself. The trouble was, he did not know how to do that in a way that felt real. He went on a bit talking about various things he had done in the previous few days to protect himself from the encroachments of other people. (My consultee told me that, continuing the metaphor in his head, he had imagined all these "other people" as mouths eating away at Michael's pie.)

What he said to Michael was, "You asked me for help but then seemed scared to pursue it, as though asking for and getting help from me would make you too needy or greedy. What was it you wanted help with?"

"I don't know—I guess to help me take care of myself. How does anyone go about that?"

The therapist said he thought the first thing might be not to attack his own fantasies and wishes for being taken care of, for being fed. "When you say, 'I mustn't want that from others,' it's obeying the family's rule about feeling: it's not rational to want something you can't get; therefore don't want it. It's like saying, 'If I can't reach that pie, I'm not hungry for it.' "

"I do lay that on myself," Michael responded. "If something's unavailable, I think it's foolish to want it. But the hole is still there."

"Yes," said the therapist. "And it's just like you said: It's right in the middle of the pie, so it affects all the pieces."

"Uh-huh. That's how I see it now, there's a big hole at the center of me, and nothing will ever fill it up. I feel scared and sad." He looked as though he were going to cry, but then he switched to talking about a situation at work: Mark, a man slightly younger than he and earning as much, was getting off too easy, and it made him furious that he could slide out of things and get away with them while he worked so hard for his money.

The therapist commented on his going from feeling sad to feeling angry. (I later wondered with him whether this switch represented a defense against experiencing the weakness associated with feeling sad and deprived or whether it was some bottom-line anger toward people close to him—including the therapist—that Michael had not yet been able to access directly.)

Michael then replied with the kind of integration that often follows on a metaphoric insight, in which both affect and some capacity of the ego to reorganize experience are released at the same time. He said, "I just realized that Mark is carrying a lot of extra charge. Sure, I feel deprived and resentful, but it's way out of proportion to him; it seems to come from much farther back."

(The therapist told me that at that point he found himself cheering inside: "He's doing his own work!" I cheered with him and suggested to him that in his therapeutic presence Michael was beginning to feed himself. I told him I might have said, continuing the metaphor of eating and being eaten, "Yes, it comes from a much older hunger.")

The themes of intense deprivation, oral greed, and the fear of incorporation and devouring that were sounded in the metaphor were made more explicit toward the end of the hour when the patient began talking about his relationships with women.

"See, I used to think that was the problem, like the missing piece of pie, but I realize now it's just part of another problem that's deeper and older. The unavailable women I've sought out at least won't devour me. I've run away from women who seemed to like me, and I've never known why."

"Does it have something to do with that hole?" the therapist asked, as openendedly as possible.

"Yes, I think so. If I really care about someone, it makes me painfully aware of that hole. I guess if I found someone who could really give, it would make me realize how insatiable I could be. I guess I'm afraid that with this big hole in the middle they'll either see it and run away or I'll end up swallowing them up."

"That *is* what you're afraid of," said the therapist. This fear of being given to by a reliable object because it would reveal the patient's insatiability and destructiveness was later explored in the transference itself. In this way, a transitory metaphor that was registered and allowed to expand became an affectively charged representation of unconscious fantasies about the self and the node for further therapeutic work.

THE THERAPIST'S ROLE IN
EXPANDING THE METAPHOR

This metaphor of the pie, homely and seemingly quite ordinary, turned out to embody a rich store of feelings and of associated insights. The therapist had been able to take in my stance as a consultant: I had helped him to realize that at most points, and *especially* when a potentially pregnant metaphor was being introduced, he did not need to "do" much of anything. Internally, he needed to be aware of the metaphorical field that was being created and then to resonate in his interventions to the prevailing metaphor without forcing. In this way, he was able to maintain and foster it. Through the therapist's heightened listening and his willingness to stay with the metaphor and unobtrusively enlarge its deeper meanings, he was actually doing a great deal to further the therapeutic exchange. In being so held and understood, the patient was able to experience his deep feelings of emptiness. As I hope I have made clear, this was not at all an intellectual exercise in word-play. The patient shortly after this session was able to acknowledge for the first time that his lifelong conscious belief that everything was basically okay was, in effect, a lie. The patient now rejected a false metaphor born out of a false self: the one missing slice. And in rejecting that older, more comforting metaphor he found one that more painfully but truly represented his fears and fantasies, the large hole at the center. The affectively charged insight represented in this metaphor heralded a change in the therapy that permitted it to become what Balint (1968) has called "a new beginning." For the first time, in asking for succorance from the therapist, the patient approached being able to face his early deep loss: that hole or crevasse that Balint has called the "basic fault." Indeed, the new beginning must address the basic fault. In this case, Michael's growing sense that through the therapeutic relationship the hole in the pie could be experienced, examined, and even partially filled was what enabled him to bring this empty core to consciousness and into the therapeutic hour.

In this last illustration, what looked to be a transitory or peripheral metaphor was recognized as a representation of the entire psyche. These are often the most dramatic and synoptic figures we work with. Sometimes they become the focal points of the entire therapy. Frequently, they shift as the therapy enables the patient to change his or her basic sense of self. It is to such key metaphors of the self and their vicissitudes that I turn in the following chapter.

CHAPTER 4

Metaphors of the Self: Changes in the Course of Therapy

The significant insights in therapy . . . are not solutions but connections—connections drawn between previously unrelated events.

—EDGAR LEVENSON, The Ambiguity of Change

METAPHOR AND ITS CONSEQUENCES

In their useful book *Metaphors We Live By*, Lakoff and Johnson (1980) make the point that for virtually all of us certain crucial metaphors serve as unconscious representations and determinants of our lives. If we experience ourselves as entrapped, experience will be assimilated to the metaphor of the prison, the walled-in cell. I want to emphasize here not only the representational but the *determinative* function of such metaphors: They not only reflect past experience but also become filters that regulate how we see our present experience and how we project our future.

A nonclinical example can illustrate the point: Lakoff and Johnson (1980) talk about an Iranian graduate student who heard the idiom "the solution of my problems" in a very different way from its customary usage. He took "solution" to be a metaphor for chemical suspension: in this metaphor, things in suspension come to the surface and recede again. The situation is never permanently "resolved." When Americans use this idiom, it has a very different meaning, one that reflects our characteristically optimistic, pragmatic worldview:

Each problem is a puzzle, like solving for an unknown in algebra; therefore, each problem must be attacked, solved, and dispatched so that one can then go on to something else. Depending on which you choose, the metaphor has different consequences or what Lakoff and Johnson call "entailments." Thus, in the Iranian student's scheme, a temporary resolution is regarded as an accomplishment, whereas in our idiom, a temporary solution is a failure. If problems by definition surface and resurface rather than being resolved once and for all, then their reappearance would be taken as a natural occurrence, not a cause for concern. The issue would become how to dissolve, or *resolve* the most pressing problems for the longest time without "precipitating out" worse ones. On the other hand, in the traditional American view, problems that recur are regarded as signs of failure and lead to asking the question, "Where did we go wrong?"

This example has important implications for the way we regard the work of therapy. It makes me think of the discouragement with which patients (and sometimes their therapists) realize they are talking about the same old things again: conflicts about assertiveness, repetitive work problems, arguments with their parents or partners, and so on. Here too, it makes a difference whether therapy is seen as moving unidirectionally and linearly—onward and upward, or as a series of zigzags. I myself prefer to think of the course of most therapies as a spiral that requires cycling in different arcs—wider and deeper, one hopes—but traversing similar ground while moving ahead.

I am not alone in perceiving the work of therapy or of individuation as a spiral. Levenson (1983) characterizes analytic work as "a helical movement (a three-dimensional expanding spiral) . . ., since on each circling of the different parameters of data, the patterning appears more extensive within each parameter and in the overview" (p. 63).

From a different orientation, Jung (1944) came to a similar conclusion:

> The way to the goal seems chaotic and interminable at first, and only gradually do the signs increase that it is leading anywhere. The way is not straight but appears to go round in circles. More accurate knowledge has proved it to go in spirals: the dream-motifs always return after certain intervals to definite forms, whose characteristic it is to define a centre. (p. 28)

The circle or spiral motif is similarly honored in T. S. Eliot's *Four Quartets:*

> *We shall not cease from exploration*
> *And the end of all our exploring*
> *Will be to arrive where we started*
> *And to know the place for the first time.*

I am reminded of a remark made by a woman with whom I'd been working for several years. She had introduced a metaphoric image of herself, her "nice-nice persona" as a balloon face, with features stamped on it. This smooth facade, without convexities or concavities—without depth, that is—suddenly struck her as both hollow and fragile. This perception through metaphor was painful to her, but it resulted in a felt experience of her persona. "I knew it before—so much of what I've talked about today, but I didn't *really* know it the way I do now," she said.

Much of psychotherapy consists in identifying previously unconscious metaphors and discovering how we unwittingly live by them. As one's sense of self changes with therapeutic work and experimental action in the "real world," these metaphors will gradually be reshaped—often without conscious effort on the part of either patient or therapist—so that they reflect more accurately a different sense of oneself in the world. Just as dreams can chart the course and progress of therapy, so can these deep and embracing metaphors. They tend to appear with enormous vividness and often do not need to be interpreted but only need to be allowed to resonate or expand. They can therefore serve as markers to both therapist and patient of the changes wrought by and in the therapeutic process.

These key metaphors will often be metaphors for the whole person, because when we look into our own psyches, we search for what unifies our diverse experience (Lakoff & Johnson, 1980):

> Just as we seek out metaphors to highlight and make coherent what we have in common with someone else, so we seek out personal metaphors to highlight and make coherent our own pasts, our present activities, and our dreams, hopes, and goals as well. (pp. 232–233)

Psychotherapy seeks to help people make more coherent and embracing reconstructions of their histories and of themselves. A large part of such exploration and reconstruction is, in fact, the search for more expansive and encompassing personal metaphors. In constantly rescrutinizing past experience and attributing new meaning to it, we are forced to come face to face with old metaphors by which we have implicitly and unconsciously lived. A large part of the work of the therapist, as I see it, is to help make those implicit metaphors explicit, so that they become available for association, examination, and reworking within the transference.

Psychotherapeutic work should also allow the patient to expose himself or herself to new life experiences (including new feelings and new insights about the therapeutic relationship) that will themselves form the basis for alternative metaphors. In this way, he or she will engage, with the help of the therapist, in the process of trying to see life through new metaphorical lenses. To the extent that this occurs, patients' self-metaphors will reflect that change. Images of constriction and limitation should gradually give way to images of expansion and possibility. Prison doors will be opened. Cramped houses can become transformed into large open dwellings, lovingly decorated. Just as dreams can be traced over the course of a depth therapy to show the rise and fall of key themes, internal figures, and self-perceptions, so can the course of a patient's self-metaphors be charted. These kinds of metaphorical markers can indicate to the therapist how the work is going by revealing how the patient's most telling experiences of himself and his world have shifted. The two case vignettes that follow are examples of this kind of metaphorical expression of psychological expansion.

HOWARD K: FROM FLOW-CHART TO ATOMS IN MOTION

A 42-year-old systems analyst, Howard K., came to see me because he "wasn't getting much out of life." Highly trained in a number of related technical fields, he was working at a job below his talents and at a lower salary than he should have been getting. He consoled himself by thinking this was just "transitional" and that when he got things in order, he would move on and up. He was also in the process of getting a divorce after a seven-year marriage.

A solidly built man of medium height, with a shock of prematurely white hair, Howard initially appeared diffident and understandably anxious in this, his first experience with therapy. He described himself as an acutely shy child who spent a lot of time alone, reading or roaming the foothills of the Santa Ynez mountains near the small town where his father had a marginally successful hobby shop. As a child, his own hobby was magic; he became very adept at sleight of hand and card tricks, but was too shy ever to put on a performance, even for his own family. He liked hovering around the edges of adult conversations or reading adventure stories or biographies of scientists, and he had an active life in fantasies in which he had remarkable adventures and performed acts of valor.

Howard described his mother as depressed and nagging and his father as gregarious, dogmatic, and ineffectual—a man who worked at a variety of small businesses but was always in debt.

Howard lived under extraordinary pressure from a tyrannical superego commanding him to fill each shining hour with productive work, to make reading lists and only read worthwhile things, to reproach himself for not reading every book he bought, to intersperse every sentence with "I should," and "But on the other hand." He approached the therapy with his characteristic attempts to "do it right," to master it through thinking and organization, and he felt frustrated about "rambling" or "not having an agenda" (topics that became central to the therapy itself).

But, paradoxically, his life's pattern looked somewhat unplanned and erratic: At age 42, he was single after a marriage that had been entered into out of duty and convention, and had had a career life that had tacked from one field to another—naval officer, engineer, systems analyst. Superficially, his life trajectory looked a bit like that of the *puer aeternus*, the eternal boy. But Howard did not have the insouciance that is typical of the *puer*. He was massively self-recriminating and fairly depressed. Underneath it all, I could see the conflict between pleasing and spiting his father, and between the desire to surpass him and the guilt attached to outdistancing him.

Howard was a man who had some difficulty playing, and it is not surprising, therefore, that it was a while before he felt safe enough with me to even begin to "play" with metaphors. About six months into the treatment, when he was beginning to trust me, he spoke with feeling about the barrenness of his life. He confided, sheepishly, that he had a fantasy that was hard to talk about. The actually quite modest fantasy was to have a special room that would be devoted to what gave him pleasure. This room (his eyes misted up at this point) would have a beautiful oriental rug on the floor, reproductions of his favorite paintings on the walls, and his stereo set and records ensconced in it. It seemed to me a very modest and easily realizable fantasy, but to him it felt as impossible as recreating the fabled Xanadu of Kubla Khan.

When I encouraged him to tell me what image his actual life did invoke, he said, with surprising directness (he usually tensed up after any such question, frowning as though I were asking him to talk in a foreign language), "My life is a flow chart." What did this mean? He went on to give me his associations: The endless routine of it, the constant need to organize, the sense of paper stretching out to the horizon. He was trapped by paper, trapped by the constriction of trying to fit everything into its proper place. He seemed to need the order, but the predictability—the *forcing* of order—was extraordinarily burdensome. He sighed often as he told me this.

I realize that an underused aspect of himself needed to be valued and honored. Despite his intellectualizing style and his wanting to smooth out the rough edges and package everything, that world of the flow chart was not where he really lived at all. When he talked about music or going to art galleries, the tension around his mouth disappeared, his voice dropped, and his large hazel eyes teared up. This man had an imaginative, intuitive side that had been insufficiently regarded and tended, both by others and by himself. So it seemed particularly important that both of us attend to the rare metaphors he did produce and that we honor them and play with them, as far as possible. (I will cite in Chapter 7 one of his metaphors that backfired because I did not appreciate that at that point Howard was not yet ready to play with his images.)

Somewhat later into the therapy he said, shyly, that he had had a powerful image of himself: "I see myself being surrounded by a huge white dome." When I ask patients to describe such metaphors in greater detail, it is with the aim of having both of us be able to *see* the metaphoric image as clearly as possible. Howard could say only that the dome was very large and very white and that he wasn't sure exactly what it was made of—maybe opaque glass. In looking at his feelings about being under this dome, he recognized that it protected him from intrusion from the outside world, and so it was safe and sheltering. But by virtue of that very fact, it also cut him off from the outside world and was therefore alienating and isolating. He was recognizing experientially what I had observed to myself theoretically: The dome was a particularly apt emblem for the nature of his defense, showing at one and the same time what it protects against and what it forecloses. The metaphor spoke to Howard's psychological condition: He was finding his isolation harder and harder to bear, but at the same time he realized how frightening it was to engage fully—with me, with a woman in his outside life, and with men as friends.

The impact of the dome image was far-reaching. Howard had been given to ruminating about how he would forget what had happened between us unless he wrote it down right away. This seemed an expression both of his dutiful interest and of his difficulty in connecting with his own experience except "through paper." He even worried about forgetting the image of the dome, despite the fact that it had meant so much to him. I said I thought that it was unlikely that he would forget this image: Because of its meaning and because he could see it in his mind's eye, that image would stay with him and perhaps even be elaborated.

Over the next few months, he did proceed to sustain and embellish the metaphor of the dome. As he looked at the image more closely, he decided that the dome, which he had at first thought was made of semi-opaque glass, was actually made of paper (partly reflecting his defense and representing a modification of the image of the flow-chart). It was, in fact, made of the pages of books—an even more explicit representation of the way he had typically approached the world at a distance. Yet, as I pointed out to him, paper is more permeable than semi-opaque glass.

In later sessions, Howard pondered, without needing overt encouragement from me, the possibilities of escaping from this dome. It was very large, he told me, but if he could only find some way to climb or soar he could easily tear through it.

At about this time—some two years into the therapy—he met

and fell in love with a woman I will call Marcy. She was the first reciprocally loving woman he had been involved with. Partly because of our previous work and his growing capacity to seek out what Kohut (1984) would call "a mature and resonant selfobject," real life now conspired with the therapy to help him see himself in a new light. He was able to be not just sexually but psychologically intimate with Marcy, to plan after a time to marry her, and to buy a house with her in which his fantasied room would become a reality—his own study, furnished just as he had imagined it.

Increasingly aware of the crippling effects of his perfectionism, as well as his problems about outdistancing his father, he was also beginning to turn his work life around. He now actively sought out the consultation work he had always claimed to want. He also came to know more surely what kind of facilitating role he was equipped by temperament to play: not to invent new products or information but to intuitively hear and translate the work of one set of experts to another. "It's as though I'm finally outside the dome and I can use it as a bridge." What had been a metaphor of isolation had become transformed into a metaphor for connection.

As we worked toward termination, Howard produced another image of himself, again a little shyly. He felt the need, he said, to represent his new sense of himself as not being static or fixed. "It's so hard to put into words, or even into pictures, but when I look at my life now I don't see myself so much as fixed in one spot, shifting from foot to foot with the old 'Yes, but's' and 'should's.' I think what I see is more, well, it's more like atoms."

"Atoms?" I asked, surprised and excited by this turn of figure.

"Yes, atoms. You know how atoms move. They move in what's called Brownian motion—it's a sort of irregular, zigzag movement as the molecules collide with each other. It seems extremely random, but there's an order to it overall." He smiled, a little embarrassed at his flight. "Well, see, it makes me kind of—kind of happy to think of myself that way."

This metaphor seemed to me the perfect analogue of increased inner freedom that vividly condensed much of our work together. It also seemed to make sense of those disparate perceptions I had had of him at the outset. Now the tacking and the zigzag need not be the random veering of his life but could be the free movement of thought and fantasy in his internal world. The idea that both order and freedom could be combined in this way represented a true synthesis that combined elements of his personality in a new configuration: The motion, the dynamism was most apparent in this metaphor, while the order was implicit rather than controlling. Howard had come to believe that the external show of order—the flow charts, the notes on the sessions, the agenda he had drawn up to talk from—were merely props. They were no longer necessary because he had found a better equivalent inside himself: a true ordering principle inside his psyche.

SYLVIA G: FROM VERY TIGHT SHOES TO SOFT, WARM SLIPPERS

When I first saw her, Sylvia G., a statuesque, blond interior designer in her early 30s, had been married for thirteen years to a vivid, forceful man whom she loved and admired. "But Thomas drives me crazy," she said in her first session. "He's so *there*, so present; there's no way to ignore him, especially now that he feels me drifting away and wants to reclaim me."

She had not really wanted to marry Thomas; she had not wanted to marry anyone, though he was clearly the most suitable of the many men she had known. She had lived at home through college and was panicky about being on her own but knew she had to leave the confinement of her parent's home. She described her decision to marry:

You see, I had nothing else to do. I had no career then, and a life without marriage was unthinkable to me. I was tired of this series of sexual encounters I'd had, none of them very satisfying; Thomas was attractive and persuasive, and I believed what I'd always been taught at home: marriage is a necessary and indissoluble sacrament. I still believe that. But the day of the wedding I felt so anxious and nauseated, I seriously thought of calling it off.

The prevailing metaphors in her treatment were spatial, and they reflected her preoccupation with tolerable versus intolerable physical distances: How close was too close? Being side by side with Thomas was tolerable, even pleasurable (literally and metaphorically); they were good partners at running their household and their occasional joint business ventures. (He was a contractor, and they sometimes worked together in designing houses.) They worked well at tasks, at something outside themselves that could engage their attention. But face-to-face was another problem. Unless Thomas turned away from her, in anger or in distraction, she felt his gaze to be intrusive, invasive, coercive. His presence, with his renewed attentions following on a trial separation and return, made her increasingly claustrophobic. Thus, her dreams were about getting out of confined spaces and into open spaces—large theaters and houses with vast numbers of high-ceilinged rooms.

Sylvia's childhood itself offered an interesting contrast of confinement and spaciousness. The family lived on a cattle ranch in northern Montana. An only child, she spent long hours by herself roaming the family's large farm. But from her birth on, her mother was increasingly limited in her activity by progressively severe angina, and the farmhouse itself was snug but oppressively confining. Her parents' gaze, too, seemed always to be focused on her. The trio was "sealed away from the rest of the world." The three of them played out a grim drama, like Sartre's *No Exit,* in which, as Sylvia described it, two stern and rigid parents scrutinized her and demanded she be good.

A metaphor that turned out to summarize this recurrent sense of confinement was that of "the too-tight shoe," which was how she early on described her relationship with Thomas. Much as she really cared about and admired him for his brilliance and charm—"No other man I've met even comes close"—she felt overwhelmed by him much of the time unless he was ill, angry, or preoccupied. His focus on her seemed relentless (as her parents' had). Sexually, he appeared to want to "redeem her" from her initial frigidity. His patience and marking of her as sexually defective but worth reclaiming was part of the feeling of confinement: He was taking charge of her in order to improve her.

A woman whose design sense showed in the understated elegance of her clothing, she had naturally turned to clothing as a vehicle for the key metaphor of her psychological situation. Together, we explored the tight shoe. What was it like? Well, it was elegant, made of Italian leather, pale colored, but the toes were too pointed to accommodate her size B foot. (Her mother used to tell her she had elegant hands but the feet of a peasant.) She had felt almost from the beginning that she was forcing herself into this too-tight shoe, hoping that it would stretch. But it had not. Couples therapy had not helped, either.

In her professional life, Sylvia experienced a far-ranging sense of freedom and efficacy; as a designer, she was unconflictedly able to be authoritative and to assert her needs and preferences. But when confronted with her charismatic and demanding husband, she experienced a kind of hobbling, as though she were indeed having her feet bound in the manner of a 19th-century Chinese noblewoman. Whatever was phallic and striving in her was experienced as deformed in the relationship, and it became clear that at least one dimension of the "hobbling" or "binding" was an identification with her invalid mother.

Somewhere into our first year of work together, after many sessions of anguish and confusion, she announced with the force of a major discovery, "A foot shouldn't be forced to fit a shoe; the shoe should be bought to fit the foot!" This truth came to her as a startling and exciting insight.

It became clearer and clearer in our work that the relationship with Thomas could not be made to work for her and that no amount of understanding seemed to change the physical experience of near-suffocation she had begun to have more and more with him as her withdrawal spurred his increasing efforts to get close. With much sadness, and to the puzzlement of a number of their acquaintances to whom she and her husband seemed to have "the perfect marriage," she decided to leave and create her own living space in a loft a friend had found for her. Although the space itself was large, she managed to segment it into small areas for sleeping, relaxing, entertaining, and even a portion that had good steady light for painting. She had not painted since she had gone to art school six years earlier but was now taking up her brush again, this time making large, uninhibited canvases. Just the sheer motion of her hand holding the brush was a liberation for her, as was being alone for the first time in her life. She felt both power and comfort in this kind of separateness.

She told me, with tears in her eyes, "For the first time it's as though I'm wearing slippers, comfortable soft slippers that have molded themselves to my foot." In her elaboration, they turned out to be not very elegant but warm and fleece-lined. They contained her feet without constricting them, so that she could finally wiggle her toes. Her feet could breathe.

In pursuing this metaphor, I wondered about the fate of the too-tight shoes. She had by then left her husband, with enormous regret but with a conviction of the absolute rightness of her choice. "I wish I could have them in my closet, to look at from time to time, but I can't force my foot into them any longer." What this meant was that she still cared about her husband and wanted to retain his friendship if that were possible, but she could not continue to live with him.

During the course of the treatment, thinking about the implications of the metaphor, I often wondered privately whether the shoe *could* have been stretched, whether with deeper analytic work she could have been helped to see that her view of the marriage as a tight shoe was at least in part a projection. We did address the fact that the difficulty in claiming and defining her own space that hobbled her in the marriage was not an isolated phenomenon but one that came up in other instances as well, when she found it hard to resist the imperious demands of almost anyone who was close to her.

But while that may have been true, I eventually came to believe that the shoe metaphor actually described a basic bodily experience. One could speculate how much of this was a construction that could be revised, but I was finally convinced that her bedrock experience of psychic comfort—and, in fact, of a joy she had never dreamed of— could not be reduced. It had to be respected.

And her decision to leave the marriage was made differently from the choices she had made in the past. It was not based on—in fact, it violated—the rigid prescriptions of her Lutheran family with their conventional wisdom and harsh "thou shalt not's." It was a truth that was based on the wisdom of the body and of her feelings. What Sylvia found in making this choice was a freedom to respond with the truest part of herself, her feeling side that had been squashed for years. Because this was a physical, visceral truth, its figurative expression took a bodily form: the foot that was constricted versus the foot that was comfortably held.

This belief was substantiated by a dream Sylvia told me near the end of the treatment. "You'll love this," she said, "it's such a *Jungian* dream." That meant that being nearly wordless and almost purely sensory, it seemed to her to transcend her own experience and verge on some mysterious "something more":

It's so hard to describe because it was just a sense of being in something, and what I was in is also hard to describe. I was walking in or surrounded by or bathed by a huge tunnel—or tube, maybe—of light. It wasn't at all confining, because this tunnel or tube was almost without border, and it was so beautiful: the light was pale oranges and greens with pinks in it, and I wanted to linger in that light forever.

The dream had an ecstatic or numinous quality that made it very moving to me as well as to her. My own private associations were to early experiences of the "oceanic feeling" described by Freud or perhaps to birth itself. It certainly seemed to include the birth canal: Was this a dream about birth or rebirth? But I kept these associations to myself. For in dealing with such a "big dream" whose thrust is archetypal and strongly nonverbal, I generally take a stance of contemplation and reverie rather than of interpretation. So we both sat there— each of us seeing her own version of the tunnel of light. I believe, based on Sylvia's increasing trust and comfort in *our* relationship, and repeated expressions of her sense that I had "got" or understood her, that the therapy had been a kind of rebirth for her. We had often explored the feeling of spaciousness versus constriction she felt in the room with me, and although there had been times when my quietness felt like the coldness of her mother, she came to appreciate the distance as being "just right" and to experience with me both a warmth and an absence of impingement. The increasing openness of her metaphors (as embodied in the late dream image) reflected the change not only in her physical setting but in her inner world as well. Attending to her deepest longings rather than the familial or collective "shoulds" represented for Sylvia an enormous reversal, and it was this change that also colored the tunnel of light. It is not clear what the future holds for Sylvia. But of one thing she is sure: If she does engage in another committed relationship, it will be based on the assent of her whole being and it will have to be a good fit.

THE THERAPIST'S ROLE IN
PROCESSING KEY METAPHORS

What does a therapist need to "do" with these embracing metaphors of the patient's psychological situation? Very little, it seems to me.

They arise from the unconscious when the interpersonal field is favorable, when the container is strong and safe. My role in these cases was to provide a setting in which such metaphors could flourish. I did this by my interest (not coercive or exclusive) in these products, by encouraging their exploration, by attending to the affect that invariably accompanies them. Metaphor often carries not only affect but insight as well, so that the therapist needs to do very little. It is more a question of attentive receptivity. I often feel I am functioning as midwife, "catching" the psychological baby as it emerges. I have more and more come to believe that if one can provide a favorable field, the patient's unconscious, acting through the ego, will do its own work.

In Sylvia's case, for instance, I could have pointed out that shoes need to fit the foot rather than the other way around. In fact, shortly before Sylvia arrived at this notion, I had what was probably a concordant countertransference dream, in which I was saying to a waiter in a restaurant, "Egg-cups must be shaped to fit eggs, not the other way round." But I didn't want to spoil the discovery I felt Sylvia was on the brink of making herself. So I let her work toward her own truth.

As for the tact to know when interpretation or further exploration is advisable and when they distract from a profound affective experience—this cannot be taught by prescription. Given a willingness to play when the patient can play, dedication to maintaining a field that is both empathic and contained, I believe that the psyche will do much of its own work.

What we can do as observers as well as participants in the process is to read these large-scale metaphors as markers both of the patient's psychological state and of the course of therapeutic work. The unyielding imagery of prisons, traps, and constraints suggests that something in the work as well as the psyche is stalemated and can occasion a further look at what is happening in the transference and countertransference. Conversely, images of increasing largeness, openness, and flexibility suggest enhanced freedom and growing individuation.

CHAPTER 5

Metaphor and Defense

Can you really see these [metaphors] as mere figures of speech when it is the figures themselves that are the active principle of the rhetoric of discourse that the analysand in fact utters?

JACQUES LACAN, Écrits

I n this chapter, I will consider both metaphors *as* defense and metaphors *of* defense: first, how metaphors that are used defensively can be worked with "within the metaphor" so as to minimize defensiveness; and second, how metaphors can reveal to us the patient's inner experience of his or her defensive situation.

METAPHOR AS DEFENSE

In the psychoanalytic tradition, everything the patient says is taken as questionable, as merely the manifest presentation of some unknown, latent, needing-to-be-disguised unconscious reality. From this point of view, as we have noted earlier in the discussion of primary process, the patient's figures of speech, like everything else the patient produces, are suspect.

For example, Caruth and Ekstein (1966) say that

> the normal or neurotic person . . . uses the metaphor by choice, in the service of goal-oriented thinking, and at an abstract level. He may choose the metaphor as a sort of alibi, a conscious allusion which is a way of implying what he wants to communicate without actually committing himself, a way of simultaneously keeping and revealing a secret. (p. 38)

They imply that these people are bent on concealing as well as revealing—a conclusion that I believe is too sweeping and is based on a view of the unconscious as a cauldron of seething impulses that one is always at pains to suppress or repress. The belief in this cauldron metaphor will itself shape how the therapist treats the products of the imagination. If one has a view that the unconscious contains more than forbidden impulses that have been repressed and that that "something more" can be illuminating, one will be more sympathetic to its products.

The Metaphoric Code

More disturbed patients may have less conscious choice in the figures of speech they use. For them, metaphor may be unconsciously driven as a kind of code to keep the threat of direct contact and communication at a minimum. So, for example, in describing his treatment of a young schizophrenic woman, Aleksandrowicz (1962) tells of how in her panic at her developing erotic transference, she shifted to a chair farther across the room from the therapist and insisted that the door be opened. For a long time, she could only express her feelings toward the therapist indirectly, through metaphor. She speculated that someone who was caring for a sick parakeet might be infected or die. The therapist responded that people who were trained and skilled could prevent that from happening. Later, she spoke of a nurse who had hugged a dying child and had gotten sick and died. The therapist, staying within the metaphor while speaking to the subtext, answered that hugging a dying child might not be the best thing to do. When she asked if a doctor would refuse a dying patient's wish to be kissed, the therapist said that "patients should be given medicine not kisses" (p. 94).

All this sounds rather cold on the surface, since we know that sometimes dying patients need hugs more than medicine from their caretakers, but I assume Aleksandrowicz was directing his interventions not at some general belief but at the specific fear the patient was presenting: She was afraid that she or he would be overwhelmed by erotic impulses and needed to be told that these would be contained. In this account, he noted that the patient could not be reassured directly any more than she could make her statements directly; but that talking obliquely in the language of her metaphor, he and she could share a nonthreatening communication. All this comes under the heading of "interpreting within the metaphor," a subject I shall say more about shortly.

Meantime, I must underline Aleksandrowicz's (1962) descriptions of metaphors as "archaic" and "regressive." I contest this notion of primitiveness, in part because it pathologizes metaphor. Some metaphors do arise from archaic strata, particularly the most primary, bodily, language-defying experiences. But we also associate figures of speech with the most sophisticated and artful use of language—a phenomenon that some psychoanalysts do not sufficiently appreciate. The indirectness of metaphor allows but does not *require* that it be used defensively. How defensive a given metaphor is depends on the context, on the psychological status of the patient, and perhaps most important, on the degree of trust between patient and therapist. A metaphor can be used not out of a need to disguise but because there is no way to express that thing directly. This happens when any or all of the following apply: The affects are overwhelmingly strong, our ordinary language is impoverished, and/or the experience being processed was nonverbal to begin with.

But of course, sometimes metaphor *is* used defensively. For example, a patient described by Shengold (1981) referred to his mother's pubic hair as her "bush." This contemptuous euphemism, says Shengold, defended against the feelings of terror and desire evoked by the sight of his mother's genitals. Several other accounts, describing fairly disturbed patients, typically children or adolescents, show us extended instances of metaphor used to defend against a more direct mode of communication which would be too threatening. In these cases, of which I give examples below, therapists have often taken the tack of respecting the defense and working with it in an extended and deliberate way until the patient could signal that he or she was ready for a more frontal engagement.

Interpreting within the Metaphor

I have already cited the patient of Aleksandrowicz (1962) who talked to him metaphorically about dead birds, dead children, and dying patients as a way of communicating her fears about her erotic feelings toward him and her need for reassurance that he would maintain the limits she feared might be transgressed. Later in the therapy, this woman could begin to tolerate more direct interpretations that went "beyond the metaphor." Thus, when she talked about dieting and wanting to lose weight, she could hear and tolerate her therapist's speaking of her wish to become smaller so that she did not have to leave the hospital and him. Eventually, more direct process interpretations could be made about the defensive nature of her metaphoric communication.

Aleksandrowicz makes the interesting point that for people who have trouble distinguishing between thought and action, metaphor may actually help with that distinction. Metaphor is a way of thinking that does not lead to action because it is more clearly "as if," a playing with possibilities rather than enacting them. The obliqueness of metaphor relieves the anxiety that would be generated by more direct communication in patients who have trouble distinguishing thoughts from actions (for example, those who feel their murderous fantasies or impulses are equivalent to murderous acts). When therapists talk to such patients within the metaphor, their anxiety is reduced. But, he cautions, this interpretation within the metaphor should not go on too long. The idea here seems to be that such interpretation is a stopgap or temporary measure, invoked only to reduce anxiety and establish trust so that the patient no longer needs to be so indirect.

Aleksandrowicz's work took off from earlier papers by Ekstein and Wallerstein (1956) and Cain and Maupin (1961), in which borderline psychotic children were treated within the symbolic frame of reference used by the child himself. Ekstein and Wallerstein found that with such children direct interpretation of conflicts often led to panic, whereas slower, more cautious use of the patient's own metaphoric currency led to the resolution of conflicts. They (Ekstein & Wallerstein, 1956) distinguish between two uses of metaphor: (1) the ordinary playing back and expanding of patient's metaphors that occurs in the therapy of better integrated patients, leading eventually to an elaboration of "meaning and intent in secondary-process language," and (2) "interpretation within the regression" for disturbed or regressed patients:

> Interpretation within the regression . . . is predicated on the assumption that the patient's ego state directly reflects the extent of his ability to come to terms with the conflict. There-

fore, communication remains within the confines of the patient's expression until some future time in the treatment when the patient himself indicates his capacity for fuller understanding. (p. 310)

This kind of communication is exemplified in the description by Cain and Maupin (1961) of the treatment of an 11-year-old borderline psychotic boy. Near the beginning of therapy, he was working at an easel, painting a picture of a dog. Suddenly, he became terrified at the spreading of the paint that was dripping down from the dog's leg. As he experienced a fear of messing and perhaps of losing his boundaries, he began to scream, "The fire is spreading everywhere." The therapist said, "But we have a fire engine," and together the patient and therapist painted a fire engine which they talked about as putting out the flames. The therapist's interpretation, following on this direct participation in the metaphor was, "It's good to have a fire engine around, even when there's no fire, standing by, in case." The child said, "Amen," and recouped from the violent disruption of his play. He continued to play and to talk in a metaphoric way about the helpfulness of the therapist (Cain & Maupin, p. 307).

Similarly, Caruth and Ekstein (1966) tell of a schizophrenic adolescent who began her therapy by talking about islands being cut off from the mainland. The therapist pursued the metaphor and, working within it, spoke of how he would try to build a bridge to the island; then, if she wanted to walk on the bridge she could, and if not, she needn't. Later in the hour, after telling her that Mexico City had originally been an island, he made the following interpretation, operating within the context of the metaphor the patient had introduced:

At first the Aztecs were isolated and alone and do you know why they were alone, why they preferred to live on islands? . . . It was safer . . . in those days the tribes used to fight each other and on an island in the middle of the lake it was easier to defend it because the enemies could not get to the island. And only later when the tribes around them became all their friends, then they slowly built bridges from the island to the mainland and after a while the islands were not needed any more. (p. 39)

Several of these writers feel that interpreting within the metaphor is especially useful with severely regressed or borderline patients in order to show them that they are heard and to enter into their frightening or shadowy world in a way that preserves distance while maintaining connection. At the same time, Cain and Maupin (1961) reflect a typical apprehension about the dangers of continued interpreting within the metaphor. They hold that because it is pleasurable to the therapist, drawing as it does on intuition and verbal play or even a kind of "magic," metaphor can have excessive allure for therapists as compared to the more pedestrian use of language. I hear in this a disturbing suspiciousness of the presumably "addictive" properties of metaphor. I contend that *any* singleminded kind of interpretation—whether singleminded in form or in content—is dangerous. Anyone who focuses almost exclusively on metaphors, or dreams, or aggression, or genetic material, or, yes, even exclusively on the transference is forcing material into his or her own template. But I feel that Cain's and Maupin's strictures go beyond that and are based on the older psychoanalytic fear and distrust of primary process. Similarly, these authors say that patients may continue to want such interaction after it has outlived its usefulness. Again, the nonlinear, nonrational use of language is treated as a dangerous drug. (I am reminded of Plato's fear of the powers of poetry and the need to exile poets from his ideal republic.) Or, to change the metaphor, patients are seen as babies who stubbornly refuse to be weaned.

The argument is made that if this mode of interpretation is used extensively it may prolong defensive intellectualizing, imposing a kind of pseudocommunication on a shaky structure. Of course it may, but not if the affect *behind* the metaphor is recognized and addressed, as it is so brilliantly in Beulah Parker's account of her long-term treatment of a borderline adolescent boy.

Extended Use of Metaphoric Code in a Borderline Adolescent

My Language is Me, Parker's recounting of this six-year treatment using extended metaphoric code, which appeared in 1962, has become a classic in the clinical literature. It is a remarkable example of working within the patient's metaphors effectively over many years until the boy himself showed that he was able to acknowledge his use of this defensive "code" and eventually to do without it.

In her comments to the treatment notes, Parker talks about how unconscious "resonance" occurs in the therapist's recognition of the patient's play on words—a resonance that permits a sharing of the feelings evoked. For instance, her own empathy was the basis for her knowing at the beginning of the treatment that her patient's theft of a carpenter's level from a school woodworking shop was a symbolic act. She made use of this symbolic understanding in the very first session when she found herself, in a kind of resonance that was not fully conscious, referring to "the level of the economy," intuiting that the word "level" would connect with her patient's metaphoric network; he quite accurately read the unconscious intent and made immediate reference back to his theft of the level.

During the first year and a half of this adolescent's treatment, the patient talked largely in what the therapist and patient later came to refer to as "code," a symbolic metaphor system in which machines or geometric objects were used as the metaphorical vehicles to communicate feeling states that were too painful or threatening to talk about directly.

Most often, at the beginning, the therapist would talk back in the "code" to show she was tracking him, while permitting the patient to maintain his defense: For example, in one session the patient had been talking about making a robot, and he said he was afraid that if the robot had reasoning power it might destroy the world. The following dialogue (Parker, 1962) ensued between him and the therapist (the therapist's remarks being given in parentheses):

> I wonder how much it would cost to make a robot? (No matter what it cost, it would be worth it if one could make such a potentially productive machine work well.) I read a story about a robot that learned to do something when it became attached to a certain man. At some point it came near to making an explosion. The man got scared and influenced it to forget everything it had been taught. (One might have to risk an explosion now and then experimenting with such valuable materials, but one could work slowly, under conditions that would keep destructiveness to a minimum.) (p. 65)

In this exchange, patient and therapist are using the same metaphoric vehicles, but the metacommunication goes on as well, like a ritualized dance or game. The players both know it is an "as if"—the therapist, from the start; the patient, increasingly as he goes along.

At other times, Parker would begin to translate. She translated the boy's speculation that an iron pipe might bend under the weight of the motor into his fears of being too much for someone (and by implication, for her) to bear. (An associated meaning about his fears of impotence was too forbidden to be interpreted at that juncture.) She took her cues about translation from him as trial borings indicating where his defenses were penetrable and where they had to be rigidly maintained. References to the transference were most difficult for him to accept at first: He ignored her early attempts to translate his talk about unstable compounds as relating to her vacation, but he was able to accept occasional translations that were less immediate. Thus he could agree that his talk about approaches to a maze was a way of speaking about his difficulty in knowing how to get close to people in general.

This young patient seemed aware that although the coded form of message he used was "partially intended to keep the other person from understanding his true feelings," it also motivated both participants to get at the emotional component of his intellectualized utterances. The boy himself said that if one communicated directly, "there wouldn't be any problem, and it's the problem that makes it interesting" (Parker, p. 99). In an hour that came near the end of his six-year, 216-session treatment, the following interchange took place, beginning with the patient's comment (Parker, 1962):

> When a person has to penetrate the code, they are bound to pick up the feelings behind it. (And if you communicate directly, they may not bother to try any more.) Yes. (That reminds me of something you said when we first started. You indicated that you had to set up conditions which would prove that a person was willing to bear some discomfort in getting close to you, so that you would be sure they really wanted to.) I suppose that's so. (p. 336)

Parker noted that this function of speaking in metaphor has not been sufficiently stressed in the literature. Analogical or metaphorical talk requires hard work to get through to the emotional component of the formulation, but she asserts that such work is richly rewarding. This appreciation of metaphor as opposed to viewing it as purely defensive is reflected in work that followed on Parker's, most notably the papers of Rubinstein (1972), Arlow (1979), and Shengold (1981).

In the hands of a practitioner as exquisitely conscious of its affective charge as Parker is, the process of talking in metaphor becomes less a defense and more a signal or opportunity. To my mind good therapy often requires if not extended immersion in metaphor, at least a willingness to engage in joint play about it. That means we must see figurative language as something other than an addictive drug or a trap. Indeed, the figures we use *about* metaphor are highly indicative: As I read the psychoanalytic literature, especially among object relations theorists, I find that over the past two decades many analysts are much more unapologetically receptive to making space for such play. The work of Winnicott especially has legitimized this view of the therapeutic space as a transitional or play space, a view I will consider in greater detail in Chapter 8.

METAPHORS OF DEFENSE:
CONFINEMENT VERSUS DIFFUSION

I would like at this point to shift the focus slightly. Now we will look at metaphor not as a way to maintain a safe distance but instead will see how metaphors can illuminate our understanding of the patient's inner experience of the self and the world, particularly what is feared and how these fears are defended against.

I am not suggesting an invariant yoking of specific mechanisms of defense and specific metaphors, although a systematic study of this relationship might be revealing. It is clear that in some general ways characteristic modes of defense will give rise to certain emblematic metaphors. Highly obsessional people, for example, may not only seem mechanical but will often think in metaphors of mechanism (machines, robots, geometries), as Parker's young patient did. The withdrawn schizophrenic patient described by Caruth and Ekstein (1966) found the metaphor of the island an analogue of her inner situation. I have observed that patients with phobic features produce metaphors having to do with enclosed and suffocating spaces or with frighteningly vast open spaces.

What all these metaphors have in common is that experience is reduced to a single dimension or template. The template has the advantage of making the world predictable and hence safe. The disadvantage is that it forces things to fit that do not really fit and hence excludes experience that a more flexible template might embrace. In short, these metaphoric templates—Schafer (1983) calls them "narratives"—both protect and deprive. They thus enable us to see the twofold nature of defense: what it protects us against and what it forecloses.

We can think of these large-scale metaphors as generic expressions that may have arisen from psychosomatic concerns discussed in Chapter 2. Reflecting back on the dimensions Fisher and Cleveland (1968) posited with respect to body image, we find that our patients talk to us all the time about the relative denseness or permeability of their boundaries and defenses. Indeed, I have had patients (especially some with eating disorders) who are so obsessed with their bodies that the body itself becomes their prison.

An excessive concern with boundaries, with sealing in, will lead to images of confinement—the prison in its many forms. An inability to create structure may lead to images of an oppressive diffusion. This raises a larger question of defense versus deficit. These overarching metaphors may reflect both. As Ogden (1986) points out, splitting starts out as a way the infant organizes the flux of experience; it may later become entrenched as a defense. Analogously, a condition that represents failure to impose structure may become actively used in a defensive way. For instance, fogginess may represent the failure to experience differentiation from early caregivers. But fogging out may also represent a retreat position when stimulation becomes unbearable. I believe that we tend to return to our psychological home base: No matter how cramped or how empty or how squalid that home base was, it is, at least, known. A patient once told me speaking about her depression that "it feels like home—a gray and sparsely furnished room, but it's a room I could walk around in in the dark, where I know every sofa and chair and every ugly knickknack." A new room might be more inviting but would clearly be more dangerous.

I emphasize here two things: (1) the importance of spatial metaphors in revealing the patient's inner space and (2) the duality and complementarity of defense and deficit, of protection and constriction, of the hated known that is so persistently sought. Within this emphasis on the opposites and the need to contain them (a central emphasis of Jungian thought), I will explore two such opposites—spatial metaphors that increasingly represent both the defensive position and the wish for the opposite that could bring greater balance and integration. Of many possible examples, I should like to focus on two generic ones having to do with extremes of confinement and of diffusion: the prison and the fog.

Metaphors of Oppressive/ Protective Confinement

Case Example: "I Am Trapped"

Metaphors of walls and traps were prominent in the therapy of a woman I saw for a number of years. Marilyn W. is a special education teacher who came into therapy some years ago in her mid-50s. She is a small, slim Eurasian woman, with her still-black hair in a tight bun. Born in Shanghai, the daughter of a Chinese mother and an American father, she had been called Mei-ling till she and her family emigrated to California after World War II, when she took the name Marilyn. Eventually, Marilyn had married, had had two children, and had taken up a career in special education. She came into therapy primarily to deal with the recent death of her 80-year-old mother. The fourth child in a family of seven, Marilyn had always felt lost in her family, as though she felt she had no clear identity in the minds of either of her parents but particularly for her mother, who seemed to her to combine a traditional Chinese insistence on rules of behavior and appearance with an almost nonexistent sense of self. "Beyond the rules, there seemed to be no one home," Marilyn told me. It was as though a mist or fogbank was held within a prison.

Marilyn's perception of her mother in some ways mirrored her perception of herself. She described her mother in vague terms: Her mother was very rigid; she was very devoted to good works, tending to the poor and sick in the extended family; she was full of rules and prescriptions. Yet at other times her mother was also vague, undefinable, looming. She saw her mother as a huge wall—like the Great Wall she had seen in her history books in Shanghai; and when I explored with her what the wall looked and felt like, she said it was high and endless: solid rock extending without visible limit. Her mother was a woman the child Mei-ling could not penetrate and from whom she received very little in the way of real attunement. Yet at other times her mother seemed more like a cloud—shifting, shapeless, ungraspable.

The alternation between the two metaphoric vehicles seemed to embody different representations of herself as well as of her mother, and to suggest an inchoate sense of herself as alternately being stubbornly entrenched and not quite there. Marilyn had felt lost in her large family, confused, watching but feeling she never quite got the hang of things. Walls and prisons have a special meaning for Marilyn because from 1941 to 1945 (the years when she was ten through fourteen) she was in fact imprisoned with the rest of her family in a Japanese prison camp in China. The experience was extraordinarily mixed for her: On the one hand, she suffered from malnutrition and the food was slops she could hardly stand to eat, and children were crowded ten to a room. On the other hand, her father was really present for the first time all the time, and the family developed a kind of we-against-them cohesion she had never experienced before. She herself became a "good mother" to the younger children in the camp, a role she has continued to play for the learning-disabled children she teaches.

In retrospect, the prison camp became a symbol par excellence of the entrapping haven. It was depressing and frightening, and yet she felt protected there as she never had at home. Years later, when the family had emigrated to California, she looked back on that time as the most clear and cohesive of her life.

The traps or prisons patients speak of are double-valenced. On the one hand the prison constricts, prohibits movement, narrows one's view, limits even the oxygen one takes in. But further exploration almost always reveals why the prison is sought. The other side is the prison as protection: It prevents the acting out of unacceptable impulses; it prevents frightening access to and contact with others; it offers an awful kind of security. I recall an agoraphobic patient many years ago who having reached the age at which her mother had suffered a psychotic depression, suddenly found herself almost unable to leave home, where she engaged in an expiatory orgy of domesticity.

She would alternately see her home as the only safe place to be *and* as a world of unbearable limitation.

For Marilyn, my Eurasian patient, traps and prisons were every-where. She might occasionally feel optimistic and even contemplate spacious vistas ahead if she looked back on her childhood and youth and realized how much freer and better defined she felt now. But if she looked at the dreariness of her dead-end job and the school bureau-cracy, it sometimes seemed she had only substituted one prison for another. In the course of therapy she came increasingly to understand how much the prisons she saw around her were actually representa-tions of inner prisons, partly self-constructed. She came to understand that the prison metaphor spoke to her felt reality but that it was not *obligatory* to see the world that way. She also became aware of the element of gain she had been getting from this metaphoric construc-tion: A trap is awful, but it is also comfortable. It is predictable and safe. You can feel virtuous when you feel you've been unjustly im-prisoned, and others will sympathize.

From being an isolated metaphor at the beginning of the ther-apy, entrapment/imprisonment became a more and more clearly sounded theme, with numbers of variations, sometimes appearing in dreams, sometimes manifesting in the transference. It became clearer eventually that what Marilyn really wanted was not to be imprisoned but to be firmly contained. For example, when I offered at one point to change her hour to a time that would have been more convenient for her, she gratefully agreed at first but became progressively anxious during the hour. When I explored what was happening, I saw that the change, far from making life easier for her, was enormously threaten-ing. She needed the certitude of a tight frame. The consistency of time, place, and duration did not seem to her at all confining, as it occasionally does to some patients. Rather, it seemed *defining*, abso-lutely necessary to the feeling of being held, as the experience of being tightly swaddled contains and protects the infant.

In the course of treatment, Marilyn's metaphor system shifted slightly: Instead of brick walls, iron bars, and prison cells, her contain-ing environment was more often described in terms of glass. She had a number of memories of looking out from behind glass at other people who were engaged in active lives that she merely observed in wistful confusion: looking through the glass panes of her grammar school at children at play in the playground; looking through the glass windows of the prison camp infirmary at her brothers and sisters. She dreamed she owned an exotic bird—a toucan, with a brilliant orange/yellow beak—that was beating against a glass window-wall, trying to escape.

The shift from brick or metal to glass suggested to me that the barriers had become more permeable, at least to sight if not to full contact. Being behind glass does shut you off from touch, but it permits you to see and be seen: Glass is an intermediate kind of barrier between the total opacity of dense, durable stuff and the freedom of open air.

As often happens between therapist and patient, Marilyn and I developed a vocabulary, a reference point that enabled us to use these metaphors—"prison," "trap," "the Great Wall," "behind glass"—as part of the currency of our therapeutic exchange. They remind me of the kind of shorthand phrases, tag-lines, and catchwords that husbands and wives develop out of a sustained common experience. These shorthand terms called up for each of us a congeries of associations born out of the therapeutic process. Thus I heard her "toucan" dream as perhaps containing a punning indirect reference to the therapy itself. One cannot fix this situation, but perhaps two can—she and I working together.

Therapy as Imprisonment

In a wonderfully vivid chapter in The Analytic Attitude, Schafer (1983) talks about the prison metaphor—or what he prefers to call the prison narrative—which characterizes many patients' experience not only of their lives but also of their analyses. The more stringently bound a therapy is, the more likely this metaphor is to surface. A treatment characterized by very frequent sessions at fixed times and with sharply observed time limits, stringent rules about payment for missed hours, the pull toward regression through the use of the couch, and the relative silence of the analyst—tends to evoke this metaphor more acutely than would a looser, less intense, or less bounded one. (But I have observed that someone for whom the prison narrative is focal can convert any setting into an Alcatraz. We have all seen our share of inmates.) Schafer's exposition of the prison narrative in *The Analytic Attitude* is sufficiently rich and compelling to justify reviewing it here. Although Schafer is skeptical of large-scale vague metapsychological metaphors of psychic structure (id) or function (projection), he is critical mainly because these are often unexamined and reified without the user's realizing they *are* metaphors. He prefers instead to speak of people acting—hence his "action language" (Schafer, 1976)—not only because it is more accurate but because such action language embodies the sense of agency that many patients have lost or have never developed.

But Schafer's skepticism about large-scale, unexamined metaphors as used by analysts or metapsychologists does not extend to the figures of speech that are used by *patients*. These he actually takes very seriously, knowing full well the power metaphor has to determine as well as to reflect our experience. He tries in practice to circumnavigate them, to look around and into them from all sides. In fact, he insists almost on a literalness of the metaphor. Schafer (1983) tells us that when a patient says "I am crushed," she may be using it in an "as if" way, but there seems to be an almost physical enactment of the metaphor: She will slump as she walks, speak in a low voice, and so on.

Accepting such a metaphor as a literal rendition of psychological states does not preclude trying to understand how the patient's experience came about and what it signifies. So, for example, the therapist can hear patients who talk about feeling imprisoned, both in life and in the therapy, as disclaiming responsibility (the ways in which they entrap themselves) even as one simultaneously appreciates this vista into the patient's inner world.

The imprisoned analysand, Schafer tells us, treats everyday realities as imprisoning and may even put pressure on others to become their guards or wardens. In analysis as elsewhere the patient is "serving time," awaiting not liberation but a verdict or judgment. He implies that a negative therapeutic reaction is fairly common among such patients. In getting better, they use their progress like a policeman's club to bludgeon themselves with the realization of how bad or how badly off they were before, how long it took them to realize something they should have known, etc. These realizations then can easily become the ground for feeling that they don't *deserve* to improve.

What I find most valuable in Schafer's analysis is his characteristic appreciation for the overdetermined complexity of thought and behavior. He reveals this in describing how people with different character pathologies can use the prison narrative in different ways. It can be used as a protection from sexual or angry impulses, it can be a hypochondriacal response to deficit, or "it may stand for an obsessionally isolated, depressively depleted, narcissistically aloof, or paranoiacally persecuted life as a whole" (Schafer, 1983, p. 266). Thus, the metaphor does not speak to any one defense mechanism or character type but depicts a home in which many different patients feel themselves forced to live. Much of their analysis, he feels, consists in learning how they unconsciously collaborate in their own incarceration.

He reveals another double aspect of the metaphor in discussing the paradox of "the happy prison." This mind-forged jail of the patient's combines at one and the same time "sensual and hostile gratification, defensive security, guilt-relieving punishment, and perhaps some vestiges of adaptation to what were experienced early in life as traumatizing experiences" (Schafer, 1983, p. 265).

Given his bent about claiming responsibility for one's actions (as well as accepting the limitations in what one is realistically responsible for), Schafer thinks of the imprisonment metaphor as looking passive but having very active elements; these include reproach and accusation, whether direct or implied, bridling at control, and so on. Perhaps, his differentiated understanding is best revealed in this statement about the imprisoned analysand's transference (Schafer, 1983): "Being imprisoned amounts to reinstating unconsciously and ambivalently every kind of confinement, deprivation, humiliation, and punishment that has been experienced, dreaded, and longed for throughout the analysand's development" (p. 269). *Dreaded and longed for!* That phrase tellingly sums up the paradox of the happy prison.

A patient, Schafer tells us, can present the prison metaphor either explicitly by complaints and reproaches or implicitly by being extraordinarily dutiful, meek, and accepting of the rules. In such a context, the analyst may in his or her countertransference become the jailer the patient perceives: He or she may become the tenderhearted jailer who cannot bear to be doling out meager prison fare and is tempted to open the prison doors and grant special privileges. Or the analyst may become the flinty jailer who responds to attempts at strikes or jailbreaks with ever stonier silence. Thus the therapist too participates and feels the poignancy of this metaphor as he or she begins to feel imprisoned by technique or stance—or by the patient.

Instead of becoming a fellow participant in this prison narrative, says Schafer, the analyst must help the patient see how deeply pervasive the metaphor is—how it informs his or her whole life and bedrock perception of self, how it gratifies as well as punishes (or in some cases, gratifies because it punishes) and what cost it entails.

In a therapy that has begun to impinge on this costly defensive position, old wounds begin to heal, and the patient experiences increasing freedom. As this happens, I have observed that the prison narrative is no longer so strongly invoked as a metaphor of the therapy or of the larger psychic situation. This greater psychological autonomy is reflected, if we are alert to the cues, in concrete images of greater spaciousness: Images of spatial constriction will gradually be replaced by images of open spaces or more permeable barriers and more flexible boundaries. Fixed dungeon doors give way to doors that slide or even to revolving doors that permit easier access to the outside world. Metal bars are replaced by wooden walls or by windows.

Sometimes life experience opens these doors forcefully, not gradually as happens in therapeutic work. A colleague tells me of a patient of his—a tall, strong man who looks like "a macho cowboy." In recounting how his wife had told him she was leaving just as he was on the verge of completing his graduate training, he collapsed in tears on the therapist's couch. After sobbing for some time, he said haltingly, "All my defenses are gone. . . . I worked so hard to be strong . . . all these years. . . . like building a tower around me . . . sitting in this cylindrical tower, building it up brick by brick . . . trying to protect myself . . . When it came time to put on the last brick on top, the whole tower crumbled, and I'm sitting here in the ruins naked . . ." He paused and added, "But, you know, it's almost a relief." My colleague reminded me of what I had already known from my study of the tower as a symbol in Yeats and Jung (Siegelman, 1987): that in the Tarot deck, the tower struck by lightning is a symbol of transformation. Or as Jung (1954) put it, "the experience of the self is always a defeat for the ego" (p. 546).

Metaphors of Oppressive/Protective Diffusion

The many metaphors that grow up around the experience of excessive permeability and unboundedness often take the form of fogginess, confusion, and emptiness. In fact they may occur in the same patients who show us their prisons, the one being a defense against the other as a kind of unconscious commandment: When the walls are too confining, fog out; when the emptiness or diffusion is too great, set up walls and bars. This diffusion that was so true for Marilyn, the Eurasian woman whom I have described above, was reflected in her perceptions of her mother as well as her perceptions of herself: Her mother was alternately the blank stone wall and a large cloudbank. In Marilyn's experience, her mother had made endless pronouncements about the rules that needed to be followed in order to keep things quiet and to save face. But behind all the rules, there seemed to be an awful emptiness that communicated itself to this child. She was someone Marilyn could not "get" and who could not "get" her. Feeling foggy was both a consequence of this lack of attuned interaction and a familiar protection against confrontation and emotional pain. As Marilyn participated in her mother's shapelessness she described the inner experience as "being surrounded with mist." You couldn't see out, but neither could anyone see you. How wonderful, you were invisible! How horrible, you were invisible! No one could hurt you, but no one could reach you.

As Marilyn began to experience this fogging out in the room with me, I was able to see and to interpret to her in nontechnical terms how fogging out repeated an initial failure of defense that then became enlisted in the service of defense. Perhaps we make defenses of what were originally our deficits. A home may be squalid, or barren, or chaotic, but it is home, what we know best and unconsciously seek to recreate.

SPACIOUSNESS WITHIN STRUCTURE:
WHAT IS HOME?

One of the questions I ask myself in the course of a therapy is: What is home for this person? Is it Rosenthal-land—the country of the Mafia (as in the metaphor of the family as a country with which I began this book)? Is it a haunted house? Is it a fog-bank? A prison? A hall of mirrors? Does it have windows and doors? How is it furnished— sparsely or richly? Is it spacious or constricted? Is it dark or light?

I am of course, talking metaphorically and inferentially. But often these images are not inferences but actual images presented by patients in allusions, fantasies, and most often in reports of dreams. Freud has talked about the house as the most regularly recurring image of the body, but since I believe the bodily experience (see Chapter 2) is largely a projection of psychological states, I would like to amend Freud and talk about the house as an image of the psyche/soma.

It was interesting to trace out in Marilyn's case her recurrent images of houses in dreams and in life—memories of her parents' large, walled compound in Shanghai, the small apartment she and her husband share (which in the course of her therapy she began to repaint and refurnish), and a fantasy of living alone in a single room, furnished with only the most prized oriental objects she owns. Her early dreams were of large dilapidated houses with no one in them and of prisons from which she was trying to escape. These were followed for some time by dreams of restored houses in seamy neighborhoods, never really her own, with shabby furniture but often with one in-explicably precious and beautiful object, such as a richly inlaid marble table—to me, a sign of the true self she was harboring, an inner richness of her unconscious that she had never sensed until then. A later dream was of a very elegant and spacious house with light pouring in but without people—a reference to her growing sense of self-worth despite recurring feelings of emptiness.

I maintain that these edifices are representations of psychic structures (and hence in a loose sense of defenses). In patients with boundary difficulties, one can trace out as the work proceeds how images of diffusion (fog, clouds, smoke, mist) will give way to metaphors of sheltering rather than imprisoning structure (houses where there were prisons, ships where there was only open sea).

I have been talking mainly about containing *structures* and the lack of them, but I think the more general metaphor system of expansion within containment characterizes many successful thera-pies. Images of weights or stones, of the leadenness and heaviness that gives depression its metaphoric flavor will yield to metaphors of soar-ing—but of soaring not at the whim of the wind but as a balloon with ballast that permits controlled flight. Defenses that once impeded movement are modulated in the service of movement. Conversely, the unboundaried begins to take shape and form. Patients talk about a new piece of territory annexed to themselves. One can see through rifts in the fogbank. An inner emptiness becomes filled as the inner house is rebuilt and refurnished now with furniture of one's own choosing—including a few valued old pieces. A safe psychic home becomes a place one can enter at will but from which one can also launch out into the larger world.

CHAPTER 6

The Therapist's Metaphors

> In the psychoanalytic situation the interaction of analyst and analysand
> is an enterprise of mutual metaphoric stimulation in which the analyst,
> in a series of approximate objectifications of the patient's unconscious
> thought processes, supplies the essential metaphors upon which the
> essential reconstructions and insights may be built.
>
> JACOB ARLOW, "Fantasy, Memory, and Reality Testing"

I f I have suggested so far that in the course of psychotherapy, the patient produces metaphors and the therapist simply tries to register and understand them or encourage the patient to explore them, I have given an incomplete picture. It seems to me that when the therapist is reasonably attuned in the countertransference, he or she will be thinking in metaphor much of the time. The question for the therapist becomes which of these spontaneous metaphoric images should be shared, and which should be held internally as a clue that awaits confirmation.

The willingness to introduce a metaphor that has not been presented by the patient varies with the temperament and training of the therapist. Many psychoanalysts would introduce their own metaphors sparingly, hewing to Freud's dictum that one does not burden the patient with one's own associations to dreams, etc. Arlow (1969a) in the quotation that begins this chapter seems to advocate mutual sharing of metaphors, but in his important paper on "Metaphor and the psychoanalytic situation" (1979) he is a bit critical of Victor's (1977) proposal that the analyst actually stimulate or shape the patient's associations by using specific metaphors from folklore, myth, or fairy tales. Arlow agrees that such metaphoric associations in the analyst's mind probably do reflect intuitive understanding of the patient and therefore represent a "commentary on the material."

Nevertheless, he (Arlow, 1979) feels that the analyst's telling the myth and explaining its import would be "awkward," though he suspects that the technique "is by no means an uncommon one, and is probably an effective one, at certain times" (p. 372).

Obviously, practitioners from other schools have different ideas about the extent to which therapists should introduce metaphors. So, for instance, therapists who are followers of Milton Erickson deal widely in metaphoric anecdotes and parables. And from a very different orientation, many classical Jungians extensively explicate the metaphorical images related to myths. Even among Jungians, there is some disagreement on the desirable extent of such so-called "amplification." According to Samuels (1985), the developmentally oriented "London school" and its adherents elsewhere hew more than other Jungians to the image of the "reticent and reserved psychoanalyst, waiting for patient material to which he might react and initiating very little not germane to the translation of what was unconscious into consciousness" (p. 199).

In my own practice, I tend to take my cue from the patient, grounding my metaphors in his or hers, and interpolating mine only on those rare occasions when they seem so compelling and so close to the material the patient is producing that they will not go away. In some cases, I make these metaphoric interpretations obliquely, believing that metaphors, like poetry, can communicate without being fully spelled out. Because I am not only interested in derivatives having to do with sexuality and aggression, I may leave only whispered, or hinted at, certain metaphoric themes that a traditional drive-oriented psychoanalyst might make explicit. In the example given in Chapter 3, when I introduced the term "basket case," I was aware of the implications not only of body damage but more specifically of castration anxiety. I also believe that it is possible to be too literal about the phallus; here I side with Lacan (1977), who regards the phallus as itself a symbol: a symbol of exchange and of power. Talking metaphorically with this patient, whose capacities for action and power in the world had been so truncated, I did not need to talk directly about penises.

Most Freudian analysts would disagree, and for one of my examples I should like to describe a metaphoric intervention used in such a traditional approach, but used with considerable finesse.

INTERPRETING BY MEANS
OF METAPHOR

Reider (1972) presents in some clinical detail a case in which the metaphor of the analyst was based on an unconscious fantasy of the patient and had its origin in the patient's concern about her body integrity. Reider describes a woman patient who came in after the birth of her third child complaining angrily about the work that was being badly done on additions to her house. Nothing was right, she said resentfully, and she regretted having begun the escalating project. Her husband, put off by her outbursts, insisted she see a psychiatrist. The analyst (Reider) made the interpretation that all this concern about remodeling represented a displacement of her fears about danger to her own body. The patient calmed down, corroborated his interpretation, and left, to return 6 weeks later, when her own sense of her uncontrollable anger prompted her to seek psychoanalysis with him.

In the ensuing treatment, the patient was consciously concerned about being slightly overweight and had a vague sense that her genitals were somehow not right, associated with a fear of having damaged them by masturbation. She could only be orgasmic by masturbation, and the erotic transference led to fantasies of being with the analyst while masturbating.

The patient had come from a very cohesive (and intrusive) family in which her father had been sexually teasing. According to Reider, the patient found it easier to be teasing—hostile or even sarcastic—than loving toward the analyst. It was hard for her to tolerate her erotic feelings toward him because she saw them as evidence of her defectiveness. Gradually, themes emerged of not being able to see or to feel and wishing not to be seen, particularly a fear of being seen in sex (she told him about her need to hide her face during intercourse).

As Reider (1972) describes it,

> The major breakthrough occurred one day when, instead of giving her the unadorned interpretation of her fear of danger and her defensive perceptual defect, [keeping herself from seeing] I said, "You know, there is a Japanese saying to the effect that a blind man is not afraid of snakes." (p. 466)

The patient agreed excitedly, and what was more indicative, she recalled an old dream from her adolescence that while she was masturbating, a lizard came out of her vagina during her orgasm. She in effect had an unconscious fantasy that she had a penis inside her which could get out and be lost if she was excited or seen to be excited. She reported a dream in which she had sewn up her vagina. This in turn led to memories of another dream dating from her childhood. When she was about five, she and her family had gone to a fair, and her father had bought her a chameleon which she loved and tied to her finger. Several days later, sick in bed with a fever, she had a nightmare about not finding the chameleon and fearing it had crawled into her body.

The patient produced memories as well as dreams in response to the analyst's aphoristic metaphorical interpretation about the blind man who is not afraid of snakes: She remembered instances of her mother's nudity and her father's near nudity. She recalled as a child pushing leaves into her ears and being told by her mother, "We don't do things like that." She also recaptured the memory of having her body in the bath washed by her mother with a washcloth, except for her genitals, which her mother washed by hand. She was remembering in effect the many mixed messages of seduction and prohibition she had received as a child—messages which the metaphor briefly and memorably summarized.

I am more interested in the metaphor and its effect than in the content to which it points, although that, too, is important. It is clear that making this interpretation in metaphoric terms led to the dramatic recall of previously repressed childhood material. What is interesting about the metaphor, apart from its respectful indirection, is its comment on both aspects of the situation: both the danger and the defense (just as her family history had contained the dual aspects of seduction and prohibition). "The blind man" refers both to the parental prohibition and the patient's repression and denial, her fear of seeing and being seen; when one can deploy this defense, one need not be afraid of things too terrible to see. "The snake" refers both to the male genital and to the patient's perceived sense of internal damage. Both the patient's defense and what she is defending against are concisely and tactfully embodied in the analyst's metaphor.

In puzzling over why this unplanned excursus into metaphor

should have produced a degree of conviction and a flood of associations that had not hitherto been possible with more direct interpretations, Reider talks about the spaciousness that metaphor can afford. This parallels the statement of Caruth and Ekstein (1966) about their already mentioned tactic of interpreting within the metaphor: "The metaphor, like the repartee of the cocktail party, permits a kind of freedom and license which is recognized by both parties to be meant and not meant at the same time" (p. 38.) Although I believe the comparison trivializes metaphor, the essential point seems to be that metaphor can hint at defenses without attacking them, and hence make them more available for patients' scrutiny. Thus, if in Reider's example his timing had been off because the patient's defenses were still too strong, she had the option of taking his comment as a bland truism, that is, "What you don't see won't hurt you." But the combination of timing and vehicle was very particularly determined: Although the metaphor was unplanned, it was not accidental because the analyst knew of the patient's interest in oriental art and Zen Buddhism. His knowledge of the affinities as well as the conflicts of this particular patient had acted preconsciously as lines of force that drew this aphorism to them, ready to be delivered when the appropriate time came. The interpretation was not a ploy but rather an example of various themes that were developing in the unconscious of the analyst as well as the patient.

Note, too, that the *form* in which the metaphor was cast was crucial. Its very impersonality—the fact that it was a "saying" rather than the analyst's dictum—offered the patient a "freedom of choice, a freedom towards activity which enabled her to break through the repression" (Reider, 1972, p. 469). The analytic ground, of course, had required patient plowing before the metaphorical seed could be received and could germinate.

In the same paper, Reider cites another example of a metaphoric axiom that a different patient could hear symbolically: Quoting from *King Lear*, he said to a patient who was complaining about a husband she had unconsciously babied, "How sharper than a serpent's tooth, it is to have a thankless child!" The patient accepted the implied analogy [your husband equals your child] more readily than she would if he had said directly (and with some implied accusation) "You treat your husband like your child" (p. 468).

In this way metaphor can open a window on the patient's psyche: It helps the patient entertain a possibility he or she is defending against. It thus embodies many of the qualities of play. (I myself prefer the metaphor of play to that of the cocktail party, since we all know that child's play can be profoundly serious, whereas cocktail party chatter is often disguise and mere time-killing.)

Although analytic interpretations couched metaphorically are, according to Reider, uncommon in the literature, he asserts that his "accidental venture cannot be unique" (p. 469). I would question, given the nature of psychic determinism, how "accidental" his metaphor was. And surely such ventures are not unique. In fact, Levin (1980) believes that the so-called "mutative interpretation"—the deliberate yoking of past and present through the experience of the transference—is essentially metaphorical.

Furthermore, the source of their power is that they simultaneously tap into many sensory modalities and several levels of cognition from the sensorimotor to the concrete to the more abstract. Levin gives an example of a male patient who had had a traumatic series of childhood losses: the death of an uncle when the patient was five, the death of his father when he was eight, and the death of his grandfather (his father-surrogate) when the patient turned 18. Apparently, any loss could feed into this man's long-defended-against grieving and experience of dependency. At one period in the treatment, the patient had had some of his clothes stolen from a laundry; he was both outraged and impelled to replace the lost items immediately (a response that reflected his typical way of dealing with loss). He speculated about getting someone to help him with this problem. Knowing that the patient's father had been a tailor, the analyst (Levin, 1980) made the following comment:

> I suggested that he needed a tailor and asked him if he knew of any way to mend the situation. This ambiguous metaphor was a reference to his major loss in childhood . . .; to his recent loss . . .; and to myself in the transference as one who mends or helps him mend himself. He recalled with vivid details for the first time a particular garment his father had made for him, just before his terminal illness. He remembered his giving it to him; and with affect he continued with new details of . . . the later loss of the grandfather . . . (p. 234)

The metaphor had brought the good father into the present in the transference. Shortly after remembering and working through this material, the patient, who had been psychologically paralyzed for months, was able to look for and find a job.

Note that all the examples I have cited were couched indirectly or aphoristically: a kind of "fortune-cookie" metaphor. A case can be made for this kind of interpretation, especially when the contents are being defended against (although if the contents are strenuously enough defended against one would question the therapeutic tact in interpreting them at that time in any case). Metaphoric communication is uniquely suited to this spacious or permissive approach. Thus, Forrest (1973) writes that because behavior is multiply determined, interpretations should not dissect out a single element but be shaped to be "multileveled, imprecise, and expertly complex, allowing the patient to choose the chief ways he will take it, which he will betray in his next associations" (p. 286). The advocacy of imprecision is somewhat unusual, since inexact interpretations have often been given a bad name. And "expertly complex" may be desirable but hard to approach: It is all too easy to be muddily complex. Although I agree in principle with Forrest's recommendations, I cannot help being struck by the telltale word "betray" rather than "reveal" used to characterize the patient's associations. This reflects a standard bias that the unconscious is recalcitrant and must be "tricked" into showing itself when the patient is taken off guard. I prefer the control mastery view of Weiss and Sampson (1986) that when the field is safe enough and the therapist has passed sufficient tests, the unconscious contents will emerge naturally, without anxiety (and often without interpretation).

Clearly, not all metaphors introduced by the therapist need be as elliptical as the ones I have cited. When infantile fears are being triggered or defended against, a more direct metaphoric translation of experience seems required. When in my own practice I experience patients as "devouring" or "empty," or when they talk about their "insatiability," the images that present themselves are of early oral need—of sucking, biting, chewing, swallowing. Bodily metaphors naturally arise in this context, and to be indirect or aphoristic at this point would be to evade the issue.

I think of a recent example of a man I had been seeing who

would tell me how wonderful his two-year therapy with me had been, how much it had helped. In the course of our work, he had recovered a number of important early memories and reestablished contact with his family to piece together a history of his first three years, which had been hazed in secrecy because he had been sent to his grandparents to live when his mother was having an affair with another man. He felt he had reclaimed a lost part of himself. And yet he felt he had to stop because otherwise he would go on forever. When I asked him to contemplate that fantasy of going on forever, he said he couldn't, he just couldn't; he drew a blank. He then spoke of his fears about his insatiability, how the thought he might go on forever terrified him, even though he got good things from me. "You see yourself as a great gaping mouth." Yes, he agreed sadly. "But then you clamp your jaws shut to protect against that feeling." This immediately produced a train of associations, moving in widening arcs from the concrete to the more symbolic. He told me that in fact he does keep his jaws clenched much of the time and that as a child, he ground his teeth in his sleep. He remembered wanting to cry at the age of three when his mother became ill and was hospitalized, but instead he held back the tears by clamping his jaws together. He was then able to think about this as a style of control and defense: warding off the tears that would spill out if he opened his mouth to take in the food he so much needed.

I believe that the *most* effective metaphors introduced by the therapist have the following characteristics:

1. They are used infrequently rather than as stock-in-trade, so that their "surprise value" does not get attenuated.
2. They are calibrated to the degree of directness a patient can tolerate and take in at that particular time.
3. They are synoptic, embracing both impulse and defense.
4. They are synchronic, bringing together past and present as relived in the transference.

But although these may be the most telling, most "mutative" uses of metaphor, other ancillary uses that are not so ambitious can also be therapeutically helpful.

ILLUSTRATING BY MEANS
OF METAPHOR

Occasionally a metaphoric image can be introduced by the therapist in order to "teach" about or illustrate a psychological problem or to indicate an alternative possibility. The explicitly heuristic or didactic aspects of any psychotherapy may be relatively slight. Nevertheless, there are often times when a single metaphoric image is worth a thousand words. One of these is when a patient describes being caught in a black-and-white, either/or position (e.g., "If I'm not perfect, I'm a failure.") Beliefs or behavior that may have some flexibility in other areas suddenly become stereotyped and rigid. Only two polar possibilities are available: black or white, flight or fight, good or bad. I have sometimes found it helpful to characterize this kind of rigid polarizing as the difference between a light switch that goes on and off and a rheostat, which permits gradual changes in intensity. Many patients find this a useful image for the rigid dichotomy as opposed to the graduated continuum.

Another heuristic metaphor has been helpful with an occasional borderline patient in the midst of a rageful affect storm that threatened to engulf us. To such a patient at such a time I have said, "All we can do right now is lash ourselves to the mast till the storm passes over." This formulation may seem to suggest that the storm is external to the patient; but it captures, I believe, the patient's experience of being possessed by an overwhelming affect, usually rage. And "lashing to the mast" conveys that I will use therapeutic containment so that we can weather the storm unscathed. The metaphor has reassured patients of my holding and of my sense that this is not the time for exploring but for enduring.

A colleague tells me about a metaphor she introduced with a patient of hers who felt stuck. She shared with him her image of him: It was as though he were sitting on the long end of a seesaw so that the other end was immovable. How would it be possible, she wondered, for him to move the seesaw to the middle position and take his feet off the ground just a little so he could see that the seesaw was not stuck but was capable of oscillating gently? (And in playing with this metaphor one might wonder about the therapist as partner, adding weight and ballast to the other end so that the two might ride together.)

These modest incidental examples of heuristic metaphors are certainly not as glamorous as the "big guns" of interpretations, but because they are visual and concrete and evoke palpable sensory experience, they become a memorable addition to the joint shorthand vocabulary of images and symbols that each therapist/patient dyad builds up for itself.

THE THERAPIST SHARES A PERSISTENT
METAPHORIC IMAGE

In working with patients I have observed that if an image of my experience of them keeps recurring I may need to find some way to share it. Such an image may occur in relation to experience that they are either unconscious of on the one hand or so familiar with that they have ceased to notice it on the other. For example, in the case of Roger F., a man I will describe at greater length in the last chapter, I kept seeing him as Meccano, the mechanical man. He was an extremely compulsive man, heavily defended against affect. His body was rigid and his talk often had a clichéd and mechanical quality: He would preface many sentences with "Very frankly" (when in fact, he rarely spoke frankly) and would make little automatic passes in the air as he said, "Not to worry" or "No big deal." I did not feel free to share this image with him until I could find some way to relate it to *his* perception or experience. Occasionally without even consciously trying I found myself introducing metaphors of heaviness and of leadenness as part of what I intuited to be his self-experience as well as my sense of him. One day after he had given a particularly heavy sigh, I said something like, "You must feel as though you're carrying around a suit of mail that seems *so heavy* sometimes. Even in here." (As I wrote these words for this book, I noticed I had written "suit of male," and I realized that the word could have been heard that way as I spoke it.) Roger looked startled at first, then he nodded. Tears filled his eyes. And then he quickly changed the subject. But I noted that that brief moment of contact caused his entire body to relax, and his associations became less managed and less stilted. Forrest (1973) makes the appropriate point—by now re-echoed in a literature that increasingly focuses on language—that

> what we are often doing, aside from providing a place with furniture for a person to go to and have some company, is *providing language* for our patients, who are having difficulties with their meanings for things, after we have listened to their language very carefully for some time. (p. 286)

A sensitivity to language is essential for a therapist—including an acute awareness of the language characteristics of others, which Forrest calls their "onymy"—their individually developed language patterns. Such sensitivity can lead the therapist to introduce metaphors at times to vitalize certain areas of deadness or repetition (Forrest, 1973):

> A good rule of thumb is that anything important, painful, or troublesome has come to mind so many times that the patient has refined his terms for those relationships into more efficient tools for the safe handling and disposal of the subject. Therapeutically, rephrasing of these terms in more lively and evocative language can uncover and enhance the emergence of feelings. (p. 286)

This "more lively and evocative language" often turns out to be the language of metaphor and simile. A colleague tells me of a patient of his who was complaining for the umpteenth time in a long analysis, about her husband. "He's like two different people," she said. "In our ordinary life outside the bedroom, he's preoccupied, inattentive, and yet aware of any criticism or even the slightest raising of my voice. Yet in bed, he's incredibly loving and expressive—almost another person."

My colleague had heard a version of this so often it was like an endlessly played record. But in trying to understand the patient's experience of her husband, he came up with an image that turned out to be very apposite: "You experience him as one of those dolls that kids have. Put it down, and it immediately closes its eyes." The patient burst out laughing, both at the surprisingness of the image and the strangeness of thinking of her complex and formidable husband as a doll. The metaphor conveyed the therapist's understanding of her experience but apparently detoxified it in some way as well. What had been threatening and troubling became ever so faintly ludicrous, and the patient told her therapist, "It's weird but, you know, I don't think I'll ever see him quite the same way again." Finding a new, unexpected image for content that has been repetitive and imageless can help patients see and feel their situation in new ways.

JOINT ELABORATION OF METAPHOR BY PATIENT AND THERAPIST

Although this is a chapter about the therapist's metaphors, I want to include an example of what I consider a "best-case scenario," a kind of "harmonious interpenetrating mixup" to use Balint's (1968) term, in which it is hard to tell who contributed what, because the interweaving is done by two partners.

I will draw my case illustration from *Forms of Feeling: The Heart of Psychotherapy* by Robert Hobson (1986), a British Jungian-trained analyst who has developed what he calls the Conversational Model. This model is grounded in the development of close relationships with patients as persons, on the assumption that what has gone amiss or undeveloped has been their capacity to form intimate ties. Hobson acknowledges his debt to Harry Stack Sullivan, as well as to Freud and Jung—and to St. John of the Cross and Martin Buber. I will report a number of the significant interchanges between Hobson and a patient he calls Freda, from an early session. Because he uses videotape for teaching purposes, Hobson is able to preserve and describe nonverbal behavior in a way that is rarely possible in the literature of psychotherapy.

Hobson titles this case material with a metaphor: "The Empty Heart." In drawing on this metaphorical expansion, I will quote extensively from Hobson's (1986) transcription (pp. 22–25). In the session he is describing Freda, age 48, tells him almost casually that her mother died the previous week. She adds that she will miss her mother but only because, with her agoraphobia, she needs someone to be with. Apart from that, she just can't seem to feel very much about it:

FREDA: It just seems to be bottled up. And I feel guilty over that, as though there's something wrong with me—that I should be crying and yet I just can't cry.

RFH: Well, I think you *are* feeling a lot *inside*.

At this point, Hobson moves toward her, gesturing from his midsection toward hers.

FREDA [with a tremor]: Inside, yes, but I . . . I just can't cry. It was the same when my dad died, and my husband. I found him dead in bed, although it was an unhappy marriage, and, er, my mother, and, er, I just can't cry. I want, I feel as though I should, but I can't.

RFH: Mm. Yes.

(In an aside to readers, Hobson comments on the importance of the well-placed, "Mm," often based, as it was in this instance, on the therapist's recalling of similar instances in his own life, and the deep affects they had stirred up in him.)

Then she says, slowly, "There's . . . this terrible empty feeling I've got inside."

The therapist notes that she has moved her hand to her chest, and he moves his hands, palms facing her, up and down, as if to say "Let's hold that feeling." When he has some sense of what it could feel like, he says, softly, "Sort of . . . empty."

Although his word is a literal repetition of her word, he gives it a different inflection: "My tone is more 'empty.' In responding, I am amplifying, not merely reflecting."

Freda choruses sadly, "Empty. Just empty." They now have in common a not-yet-fully articulated but deeply felt bodily image. And Hobson finds that his right hand has moved over his heart.

RFH: You put your hand about here.

FREDA [Freda moves her hand to her heart]: Just about here. Emptiness.

RFH: Mm.

"I pray," he writes "that the 'Mm' expresses sympathy—a feeling-with." And he adds,

I seem to hear the first chord of an emerging theme—a body-word metaphor "empty heart." The "commanding form" of a symphony can be suggested by the first phrase of the first movement. . . . We speak at the same time. A meeting is disclosed. Alone and together looking into a void.

By experiencing the reality of that shared body-image, Hobson (1986) is able to make an interpretation, which he describes much more modestly as a "hunch":

RFH: Let me make a guess . . . er . . . I think that there are times . . . when you feel bad . . . that you can't love people enough.
FREDA: That's just it.

Her response is given with enormous feeling; what her heart was empty of is, indeed, love. And she later goes on to talk of how she feels guilty about this emptiness, feels she's not normal, can't cry and thinks she should be able to.

But as she talks, she moves her hands in a way that suggests to Hobson that she is offering something to him. He feels he is slow to understand the language and vague in his reply. In responding to her statement that she cannot seem to show love, he says:

RFH: No, but you were wanting to show something then, with your hands.
FREDA: Yes, I want to. I want to show them love and yet I don't feel love *here*, and I know I should do. . . .

Freda then places her hand again over her heart, reinforcing the metaphor of the empty heart in her gesture.

Something important has been created by this careful moment-to-moment metaphor building, through words and more importantly through the *music* of the therapeutic exchange. This music derives from tone of voice, facial expression, and preeminently in this case, gesture. Later in the hour, these moments of communion through shared metaphor enable Freda to see Hobson suddenly as looking like "Dad" and to weep for her father for the first time. This change occurred because a deeply attuned observer was able to supply a resonant body metaphor.

Indeed, this kind of communication is contrasted by Balint with the communication of "insight": he speaks of insight as having to do with "seeing" or "standing"—activities that can be performed at a distance or alone. Object relationship, is by definition (Balint, 1968), interactive and

more often than not, is created and maintained also by nonverbal means. . . . In contrast to "insight", which is the result
of a correct interpretation, the creation of a proper relationship
results in a "feeling"; while "insight" correlates with seeing,
"feeling" correlates with touching . . . (pp. 160–161)

It's no accident, then, that Hobson's (1986) book should be called
Forms of Feeling, and that his sensitivity to gesture and to psychologically touching the other should be so paramount. This is
another way to look at embodiment: It goes beyond the classic Freudian modes and zones to a therapy of *metaphoric affective contact* that
speaks through the body's gestural language and is felt in the body's
inmost places.

METAPHORIC IMAGES
AND THE THERAPIST'S
EMPATHIC UNDERSTANDING

I want to go now from the therapist's deliberately introduced
metaphors to something larger and more mysterious: the metaphoric
image the therapist allows to expand in himself or herself by being in a
mode that is just the opposite of interpretive. This is Freud's "freely
hovering attention." It is this receptive and dreamy state that Keats
attributed to the poet when he talked about "negative capability"—
the ability to lose oneself in ambiguities without seeking their resolution. It is the state in which, I would guess, we spend much of our
therapeutic time. In this almost meditative state, our unconscious
resonates with that of the patient to produce sensations, fleeting
impressions, memories, and fantasies. Many such impressions are
scarcely above the level of consciousness and are ignored. But when
the therapist's readiness to experience these multisensory images
matches the patient's charged affective state, a kind of "new understanding" of the patient's situation becomes possible. We are,
perforce, allowing ourselves to know what our patients feel, either by a
kind of empathy or by being inducted into experiencing what has been
placed in us through their projective identifications.

Let me give an example. Carl W. was a pale, slim 45-year-old
man who had retired from a career in market research, and had left a

ten-year marriage and found himself unable to move on either in work or in love. What puzzled me about Carl was how little overt despair he acknowledged. In fact, his affect was rather bland. He seemed somewhat dazed and out of phase: The words and the music of his discourse simply did not jibe. He would repeat in a perfectly even monotone the talk that had been fashionable in the 1970s—so much so that I felt caught in a time warp—about how he was an "intimacy junkie," a "people person." Yet my experience of him was that he was utterly disconnected both from his own feelings and from me. He had been coming to see me for about 6 weeks, and I became aware that I felt unusually sleepy during my 2 o'clock hour with him—a feeling, I realized, I did not have with the people I saw at 1 and at 3. This was not boredom: It felt much more total and debilitating, like a drug-induced lassitude.

One afternoon, sitting there and listening to him talk at me or waiting during his silences, I had an eerie fantasy: We were both divers, we had dived far below the surface, and our oxygen lines had snapped. Submerged and becalmed, we could not really talk to each other. Our movements were dreamlike, slowed down, as though we were suffering a narcosis.

The fantasy was so vivid that I knew I had to give it room. I realized that this extended metaphor was an internal cue, an induction in me of something that belonged to the patient. This sensorimotor image and the lassitude and isolation it evoked forced me to experience directly—not through words or through the intellect—what the world was like for *him*. Having been forced, or having allowed myself, to experience his world, I was able to feel how totally becalmed and alienated he felt. I did not in this case share this image with him, although at a later time I might have done so. What seemed important to me at that point was that my countertransference shifted as a result of this experience: Through a kind of participation, I had felt some of the distressing paralysis that underlay his bland exterior. I had understood it not just in my head (as one might in formulating the hypothesis that his manic defense was covering depression), but in my entire body. This kind of total—if temporary—emergence in the experience of another changed the therapeutic field in which we moved. Whenever a therapist is suffused by such a living metaphor, the therapeutic encounter can change dramatically without a single interpretation being offered or, indeed, without a single word being uttered.

THE METAPHORIC RELATION TO THE OTHER: TRANSFERENCE DISTORTIONS AND EMPATHIC IDENTIFICATIONS

In order to pursue the metaphors implied in empathy, I need first to talk about the metaphors implied in transference and countertransference. In the symbolic enterprise of psychotherapy, the major metaphor is undoubtedly the transference, whether it is examined or unexamined, strong or weak, positive or negative. And it is a metaphor (e.g., You are my mother) passionately and blindly held at times that needs to be converted into a simile: "You are like my mother in these ways," or perhaps even more accurately, "The feelings I have been experiencing with you are very like the feelings I had when I was tiny and my mother turned away and left me to cry."

Conversely, that part of the therapist's countertransference that is not usefully informing the therapist about what the patient's experience is or has been like—that is, the so-called neurotic countertransference—is also a kind of metaphor or symbolic equation: The therapist is experiencing the patient as a significant figure in his or her own life (mother, father, child, savior, mentor, acolyte). These metaphors, too, need to be made conscious and worked through, in consultation if necessary.

But while metaphor can represent distortion and false equations, it can also be a source of understanding and recognition. This is as true in therapy as it is in ordinary life. I agree with Beres and Arlow (1974) that the therapist's empathy is in essence an *oscillating and temporary identification*. It is a fleeting sense of "In this moment, I am you." Empathy, I have found in supervising and consulting, is limited by the range of the therapist's inner development. The more complex and differentiated the therapist, the more he or she can empathize with different kinds of patients. But there will always be some people so different from us that empathy becomes misguided, and one realizes that one cannot know what it is like to be the other, even in the moment.

I am thinking, for example, not of a patient but of a hyperfactual colleague who confided to me how out of place he felt in taking a workshop in dream interpretation. I volunteered what I thought was an empathic remark based on my only experience of having felt like the class dunce. (It was when I had taken a course in Yiddish and found that everyone else in the class had some special knowledge—of German, of Hebrew script, of Yiddish itself—that I did not possess and that exposed me to the experience of feeling stupid.) So I said to my colleague, "You must be feeling awful." Perhaps this was empathic at some level, but he had to deny it and to assert that he now was clear that dream interpretation was not his thing. For this man coolness and a cognitive response would have been perceived as more empathic. I had been unable to put myself in his shoes, perhaps because his shoes were so unlike any I could ever wear. But the interchange was informative. I now know more about the defenses he uses to preserve his self-esteem and handle his discomfort, including the discomfort of being the recipient of sympathy. So I suppose that if "empathy" is partly cognitive, my empathy for him was refined by this encounter.

Much of the empathizing we do as therapists is accurate and is based on the universality of deep human experiences of sorrow, despair, rage, joy, and love. As Schafer (1983) puts it, "Unconsciously we are all members of an endangered species" (p. 47). Patients for whom we cannot make that temporary equation, "I am you," are those we will have the greatest difficulties working with. Yet I find that even those patients who initially seem to repel empathy often become more appealing as I work with them. Understanding breeds empathy, empathy breeds understanding and a kind of uninvested love. Cynthia Ozick, the novelist, in her essay on "The Moral Necessity of Metaphor" (1986), has said it far better than I can:

> Through metaphorical concentration, doctors can imagine what it is to be their patients. Those who have no pain can imagine those who suffer. Those at the center can imagine what it is to be outside. The strong can imagine what it is to be weak. Poets in their twilight can imagine the borders of stellar fire. We strangers can imagine the familiar hearts of strangers. (p. 68)

CHAPTER 7

Pitfalls in the Use
of Metaphor

*A superstructure of interesting images (which was temporarily effective)
had been built by the patient's and analyst's joint enthusiasm, but it
lacked solid foundation.*

ALFRED PLAUT, "Reflections about Not Being Able to Imagine"

*"When I use a word," Humpty Dumpty said, in rather a scornful
tone, "it means just what I choose it to mean—neither more nor less."*

LEWIS CARROLL, Through the Looking-Glass

*. . . the problem is not metaphorical thinking as such, but rather
the degeneration of such thinking through literalization in which
enlightening comparisons are reduced to identities and "live"
metaphors to "dead" ones.*

DONALD CARVETH, "The Analyst's Metaphors"

S everal kinds of pitfalls confront the therapist with respect
to metaphor. One danger is the over-reliance on metaphoric images and excessive zealousness in their pursuit. The other
and opposite shortcoming is the failure of the therapist to recognize
the subtle or implicit metaphors embodied in the patient's everyday
experience, including the experience of the therapeutic interaction. I
will address both of these problems in this chapter, as well as the
problem of the literalizing of metaphor in theory and eventually in
practice.

OVERVALUING METAPHOR APART FROM ITS CONTEXT

Although I have written this book to highlight the primacy of metaphor, I am obliged to point out that, like any other component of the therapeutic process, metaphor can be misused. Metaphors *can* be used defensively by the patient and by the therapist, giving an illusion of mutual play when in fact, only a semblance of play is taking place. So, for instance, a patient of mine whom I saw for two years and who then returned after a year's break to work in a deeper way, stopped herself in the beginning of a metaphor. She was saying, "I feel like a rag doll" when she interrupted herself to comment on her own process: "No, I don't want to say that." When I asked her why she had cut herself off in the midst of that figure, she said, "I was aware that I was trying to please you a lot of the time by drawing on our common interest in literature and by using metaphors that I knew you would appreciate. I don't want to do that this time. I'd rather tell it straight if I can."

She sounded a sobering note for me. I think a therapist cannot afford a systematic bias in his or her attention. Preferential treatment for *any* kind of material, be it dreams, transference manifestations, defensive operations, or metaphors—is loading the dice and departing from the ideal of unencumbered and unbiased attention. I am concerned about therapists who are only interested in dream material; or those who hear everything as only manifestations of the transference; or those who are able to register only sexual and aggressive impulses or only derivatives from early development. Becoming aware of one's own bias in any of these directions allows one to correct for it.

With respect to metaphor, this bias in attention can reveal itself in seizing upon every instance of metaphor no matter how casual or inert and exploring it; or in forcing an unready patient to play.

Climbing Every Metaphoric Mountain— and Molehill

Perhaps what I have said above seems inconsistent with my statement in Chapter 3 that valuable ore may flash out from even the most inert metaphor. The issue with regard to the interpretation of metaphor is one of degree and of tact. Interested attention is one thing, zeal is another.

A case in point is a paper by Voth (1970), "The Analysis of Metaphor." Voth's thesis is that in periods of intensity, the patient may introduce implicitly metaphorical words and phrases that stand out from his typical language style. Voth (1970) holds that these figures "are particularly susceptible to analysis because resistance is low at the moment they are spoken. The results of such focused analysis, if properly timed, lead directly to the deepest roots of the personality" (p. 621) and provide links to the transference and the patient's character structure and history.

I have no quarrel with this point of view. But Voth's actual case examples conjured up for me an image of the analyst as sleuth with magnifying glass, relentlessly teasing out every potential vestige of metaphor. Voth does add that the examples he gives are taken out of the context in which the usual analytic techniques of dream analysis, clarification, transference analysis, and interpretation are used. So it may be that his emphasis appears more onesided in print than it was in practice.

Favoring a kind of active or focused analysis, Voth (1970) writes, "the patient should always be asked to associate to his metaphor" (p. 621), which often yields associations different from those intuitively suspected by the analyst. Always? In the absence of strong contraindications, Voth actually advocates interrupting the flow of associations (or getting patients to reflect on them later) to associate specifically to what they have just said. He claims that the treatments in which this more focused intervention were used probably proceeded faster and were more thorough than others. He finds that the hours in which metaphors have been analyzed are particularly rich hours.

I find this too, but in reading Voth's case examples I felt that this kind of steady focused intervention could seem to a patient like badgering. He tells of a woman patient who had identified with her father and with a phallic mother incorporated as a fierce superego; the patient simply deluged him with words. Voth says that in order to keep from being rendered impotent, he had to "'fight back' psychoanalytically" by focusing on her metaphors and by demonstrating that she could not dominate the treatment. He says that when she began an hour describing the headache she had had at the end of the previous hour as "big and beautiful," he asked her to give her associations to "big and beautiful." As the reader might predict, the well-schooled patient associated to her husband's penis. When she then went on to talk about her daily life, the analyst brought her back to seek further meanings in her metaphor "big and beautiful," and she said that *she* would like to be big and beautiful; this expressed wish confirmed the analyst's sense that her chatter was a way of dominating him. When she talked about wanting communion with her husband, he asked her to associate to communion, and so on.

In another hour, she talked of being connected to her mother by a thread and beginning to become more attached to the analyst by a "string." When he noted the change of metaphor, the patient acknowledged the change with surprise and wanted to change the topic but he asked her to associate to string, whereupon she then produced "G-string . . . tampax expanding when moist . . ." The analyst moved in quickly, noting how she had transferred her wish for a penis from her husband to him; he added that because of this envy she could not compliment her husband and she was competitive with him.

Perhaps it is the tone of blame and of utterly knowing analytic superiority in this account that colors my negative reaction to it, not to mention the single note about the penis-envy of women patients that has been sounded all too often by traditional male drive-theorists. Patients can be "taught" to produce certain material, to dream in certain ways, to produce images of body anxiety if that is what the therapist implicitly requires. In the living context with a full range of cues (facial expression, gesture, tone of voice), this may have been a less judgmental interchange than it appears here. My association, however, is to the "The Taming of the Shrew" and the struggle for dominance between Petruchio and feisty Kate. The issue is: Who will have the upper hand? One can get patients to comply, as Petruchio did Kate, "for her own good." And in this mode one *can* use metaphors as weapons. I strongly believe, however, that the means of therapy must be consonant with its goals: Anything that approaches prodding is an intrusion on the patient's autonomy, and "speed-up" tactics seem utterly out of place. There is, after all, such a thing as therapeutic tact.

What is most distressing is Voth's implication that therapists who do not agree with his approach are "troubled." "I have regularly observed . . .," he notes, "that the style of treatment just described is unacceptable to troubled therapists who will generally find the quickened pace of the treatment unpleasant" (p. 619). This seems to me reductive and unfair.

"Forcing" a Patient's Metaphor

I can understand how easy it can be to get carried away by a given metaphor—particularly when produced by a patient who has heretofore been sealed off from his or her imagination, who produces few dreams or fantasies, and who lives life in the realm of the concrete. I overreacted in this way, I feel, with Howard K., whose metaphors of self I have described in Chapter 4. Howard first approached the metaphoric about six months after we began working together by telling me one day that he was dissatisfied with himself and his life, that he was tired of living on the periphery, vaguely thinking about how he might make his life more exciting but unable to realize his fantasies. He wished he were different, he wished his life felt like—he paused and groped for the image—"like a jar of jellybeans." In the gray sky of abstract language I had heard from him thus far, the image stood out like a rainbow. Experiencing the delighted surprise that for me signals something important in the interaction, I asked him to tell me more about the jar of jellybeans. He complied in a desultory fashion that seemed almost to negate his ownership of the metaphor. I did not choose at that point to interpret his response, so I simply let the image go.

Several sessions later, when Howard again expressed the wish for some excitement and play in his life, I recalled for him his "jar of jelly beans" metaphor and asked him again to tell me what it made him think of. His reply was lackluster and dutiful. "Well," he said, "I don't know. I guess jelly beans are colorful. And—maybe they're all the same shape but they'd give you the sense of variety if you saw them all together." I said, (feeling as I did so that I was coaching him in a game of Twenty Questions), "They're usually connected with children." "Yes," he agreed halfheartedly. Patients eventually teach you what you need to know. At that point, I did begin to realize that expanding this metaphor was *my* agenda, not his, and that *that* was why it was not working. So I shifted to talking about that process—about his dutiful if grudging desire to please me. This desire, he could agree, had characterized most of his dealings with authority figures, to whom he was overtly respectful while often secretly furious at the seemingly irrational demands they put on him. I could interpret how I had just become such a figure for him.

We did get some mileage from this encounter after all. And this interchange underlined for me how essential it is to scrutinize the interactional *field* in which a patient's metaphor is embedded. It reminded me that I must not assume that simply because a metaphor is produced, the patient and I are operating in what Langs (1979) has called a Type A field and Goodheart (1980, via Jung) would conceptualize as a "secured symbolizing field."

It was clear that Howard and I would have to work through his feeling of being forced to perform by me as he had felt forced to perform his magic tricks by his father—in order, as Howard saw it, to make the father "look good" to the audience of admirers, without regard for the agony his shy son experienced on these occasions. Only after working through these experiences in the transference, did Howard feel secure enough to engage in true imaginative play. It was then that he produced the image I described in Chapter 4 of seeing his life as a flow chart. This image, unlike that of the jelly-bean jar, was accompanied by affect—in this case, a palpable despair. It was the *affective* connection that made it truly his. He subsequently went on, as I have recounted, to produce spontaneously the self-metaphor of the paper dome and eventually the exhilarating image of "atoms in motion." I feel that the image of the jelly-bean jar was actually a prefiguring in more structured form of the "atoms-in-motion" metaphor that Howard ended with: The color and variety of these candies (they are shaped like eggs and are associated with oral gratification and with Easter, the time of resurrection) heralded what needed to happen in his life and in his therapy. And, in fact, in the course of treatment, he fell in love and married a woman who was much more giving than his first wife, and he grew more alive to his own possibilities. In some ways, the "atoms-in-motion" metaphor embodied greater freedom than the abortive "jelly beans in a jar," because the need for containment was less, and the sense of move-ment greater, along with a confidence that atoms in motion did not mean mere randomness but was in fact the principle of all matter.

It was not my understanding of the possibilities of his figure of speech that was faulty, it was my redirecting him to it in a way that felt to him at the time like an onerous assignment. A therapist must learn when to back off gracefully and when to use the fallout from such encounters to advance the therapeutic interaction. Forcing will not work.

My dictionary defines "to force" in its horticultural usage as "to hasten, as in growth or productivity, by artificial means; as, to *force* bulbs." What works for fruit and flowers does not work so well for people—especially for people struggling to finding the rhythm of growth in their own season. Therapeutic growth can be fostered but not forced. This brings me to the larger question of what it is that one must foster, or—to change the metaphor—how to distinguish be-tween fool's gold and the true ore of the symbolizing process.

A Non-Forcing Approach to Patients Who Cannot Imagine

I want in this context to refer to "Reflections about not being able to imagine" by Alfred Plaut (1966). Plaut is an analytic psychologist of the London group of Jungians, which is closer than classical, Zurich-trained Jungians to psychoanalysis in its emphasis on early develop-ment, reconstruction, regression, use of the couch, and so on. Many Jungians of this school, whose main founder is Michael Fordham, have drawn on the work of Melanie Klein, as well as the British middle school of object relations theorists. They thus form interesting links with psychoanalysis and find common cause with "independent" figures like Charles Rycroft, who has broken his ties with the psy-choanalytic establishment. Indeed, the last part of Plaut's paper, which does not concern us directly here, addresses the rapprochement between the ideas of "psycho-analysts and some analytical psycholo-gists" (i.e., Jungians).

In essence, Plaut (1966) contends that "the capacity to imagine constructively is closely related to, if not identical with, the capacity to trust." Furthermore, this capacity (trusting *and* the consequent ability to imagine constructively) is "severely disturbed by defects in early relationships" (p. 113).

Plaut warns that excessive reliance on images (whether through dreams or through associations) can lead therapy into a blind alley unless they are analyzed in the context of the therapeutic relationship. He (Plaut, 1966) illustrates this premise by giving a case example that had occurred many years earlier, when he was practicing

> what I would now call impact by image-psychotherapy . . . [in which] the therapist relies on imagery borrowed from a variety of sources (e.g., mythology and religion) which *appears to be* appropriate to the patient's problem. The impact of this may be impressive to the patient and thus convince the analyst that he is on the right track. But the effect is often fleeting . . . its appeal resembles that of magic. Integration is thus neglected. (p. 120)

The recantation will have more resonance to Jungians than to classical Freudians, since Jungians have more typically tended, following the practice of Jung himself to expand or "amplify" in mythological terms the dream images produced by patients.

But even for therapists who do not actively amplify metaphoric images, Plaut's warning is important. What he says about this early patient was that he had excited the imagination of the patient who seemed to absorb his analyst's amplifications and suggestions with gratitude. Negative transference did not show itself. But Plaut later learned that the therapeutic work had been merely pleasurable window-dressing; it did not hold. Plaut (1966) writes with candor:

> Only later did I learn that his [the patient's] life was in a complete mess which it would have taken blind faith to regard as unavoidable and all to the good, i.e., in the cause of the development of his personality. My revised practice is to analyse the obstacles in the way to ego-development. (p. 121)

This revised practice entailed: (1) exploring in detail (presumably through reconstruction and reliving in the transference) what went amiss in the patient's development and (2) simultaneously working to establish the patient's capacity to trust a good inner object, based on the relationship to a trustworthy "good enough person," that is, the analyst.

Plaut concludes that without such painstaking work, "a super-structure without foundations can or even will result from joint enthusiasm about interesting imagery . . . which may not be firmly enough linked with the ego core" (p. 120). These images can sometimes distract from the what is after all the *central* metaphor of the therapy: the relationship as experienced in transference and countertransference.

UNDERVALUING METAPHOR: THE THERAPIST'S FAILURE TO IMAGINE

The Mistrust of Metaphor

The use of metaphor has inspired a chorus of naysaying voices, echoing throughout the eons back to Plato, who wanted to exclude poets from his ideal republic because of their attempts to dazzle and deceive. Although Freud himself was a brilliant user of metaphor, he remained skeptical about the truth-claims of the arts because of the presence of illusion in them.

For now I want to focus on the undervalued metaphor in clinical practice. Schafer (1976) urges that when we talk to patients we use what amounts to "ego talk," verbs in the active voice that imply a whole person as agent (Not "Part of you wanted to do this, and part of you felt afraid," but rather "You wished to do this while at the same time you feared you could not.") A commendable recommendation, but one that has its limits: I agree with Ogden (1985) who says that Schafer's language is the fully articulated language of the depressive position—the stage at which a person is capable of subjectivity, compassion, guilt, and the desire for reparation. At the more primitive level of mental function in which our borderline patients spend much of their time and all of us if sufficiently stressed or deprived spend *some time*—the metaphoric constructions "I was possessed," "It overtook me," accurately reflect their inner experience. The therapist can use action language, but it seems to me that he or she must respect the fact that such language in a patient lacking in ego development may fall on deaf ears. In fact, the whole thrust of therapy or analysis with such patients may be to develop enough trust in the therapist to permit the freedom to step aside from one's enmeshment in inner experience and see that there is another way to look at things,

— 125 —

that a metaphor one has constructed can be remade. But long therapeutic work must proceed before patients functioning primarily at this earlier level can be brought to see how their metaphors limit as well as represent their experience. A therapist can continue to address such a patient as a whole person, but it may take a very long time until the patient can feel substantial enough and have enough observing capacity to begin to examine the ground of his or her metaphors.

A middle position can be helpful in this regard. By couching the metaphor in terms of the patient's psychological experience, the therapist allows it to stand as an expression of that reality while still noting its as-if quality, (e.g., "You felt as though you were totally seized and overcome, caught in a vortex").

Unlike more "concrete" therapies of the conscious that have to do with changing specific behaviors or specific cognitions, psychoanalytic therapy and analysis demand a metaphoric or—as I shall later show—a symbolic way of seeing the world. In this respect, the therapeutic and poetic enterprises are consonant. Marianne Moore, in her poem on poetry, talks of the poet as someone who can create "real toads" in "imaginary gardens." I take it that by this she means that the garden as a containing universe is so brilliantly imagined that all its denizens seem real, and we therefore approach the poem (or the novel, or the play) with what Coleridge called "the willing suspension of disbelief" and with Jung's respect for the reality of the psyche.

Analytic therapy is similar, but perhaps reversed. The therapist—and through him or her, eventually the patient as well—has the faculty of seeing the "imaginary toads" in the "real gardens." That is, of seeing the metaphors implicit in material that appears to be anything but metaphoric. It takes no great gift to recognize as symbolic a dream image or a deliberately introduced figure of speech that heralds itself and trails its train of significance along with it. But what about more subtle or embedded figures? What *else* is this patient talking about when he talks about his friend's baby who is old enough to change his own diapers but not old enough to do without them? Is this big baby himself? Is he proud of his mastery, or ashamed of his slowness? Or is the paradoxical combination what troubles him? The very act of making meaning is tied up with seeing the metaphorical extensions of what we are talking about. These extensions are rarely single or linear. They are more like a web of complex and inter-connected meaning that spreads out from everything one can visualize in the course of a therapeutic hour. Freud said that sometimes a cigar is only a cigar. But literalists see a cigar as always and only a cigar. Such literalists make difficult patients and limited therapists. But cracker-barrel symbolists, on the other hand, for whom a cigar is always and only a phallus (manifest content A always and only equals latent content B) are robbing potential symbolic experience of its richness. We ought to take an intermediary view. Sometimes, as Freud said, the cigar is best taken as only a cigar; but often it is better understood as something else, and the something else may not be reducible to one symbolic equivalent.

The Therapist's Failure to Imagine

Let me give an extreme example of a failure to imagine on the part of a therapist who was my supervisee. She had just begun a year's training in a non-degree-granting extended education program offered by a local training center for therapists who wanted to strengthen their clinical skills. For a time, I worked as a supervisor there.

My supervisee, a woman with a degree in counseling from a local university, presented to me in supervision the case of a female patient who had been raped. Some months after beginning to see the patient, the therapist, to suit her own convenience shifted their meeting place for one session from the agency office where she worked part-time to her private office in her home. She told me about this change after the fact, and when I tried to show her how the patient might see this shift as a either a metaphorical seduction or a metaphorical rape, the therapist steadfastly held to the view that I was making too much of it. She told me that the patient had taken the change of meeting place in stride and had even been pleased by it. In recounting the process of the hour, the therapist indicated that the patient's associations had returned to the rape, which she had not talked about for some time. The therapist could not see that these associations were derivatives of the unconscious fear the patient experienced in this dramatic rupture of the frame. This kind of response represented a blatant failure to see the symbolic implications of her own and her patient's behavior.

Between the Extremes of Forcing and Blindness: Respect for Overt and Implicit Metaphors

I have cited this extreme example of therapeutic obtuseness because it highlights what is often much harder to see when it occurs in smaller, more typical ways. Apart from making conscious what was unconscious, our profession requires respect for the symbolic possibility of *all* discourse, not just discourse that clearly heralds itself as "METAPHOR" in flashing lights. Our inability to see the hidden or implicit metaphors can prevent patients from enlarging the meaning of their own experience. To the extent that psychotherapy or analysis is an interpretive art and not a science, what we foster in our patients is an increased freedom to construct and reconstruct meanings so as to arrive at a fuller, more complex, and, in some sense, a more affectively true rendering of their experience. This is a kind of playing with one's life history.

Patients cannot be helped to do this reconstructive playing with their own narrative unless therapists themselves know how to play. Winnicott has said that the therapist who cannot play is unfit for the work. We need to remind ourselves that most if not all of what patients tell us can be heard on a metaphoric level (and indeed every time we translate from the patient's life experience to the transference or vice versa we are performing a metaphoric operation). By hewing to the metaphor we are conveying a message to the patient: "The lived truth of your experience need not be 'either/or' or 'nothing but.' The 'truth' most often turns out to be 'both/and.' " The therapist is both an old object and a new object. The manifest content—of a dream, for example—is not unreal and irrelevant, but part of the complex meaning of the dream. To believe that only the depth, the unconscious, is real is to slight the contributions of the conscious ego. Conversely, to stick at the surface robs experience of its deeper significance. It seems to me that a respectful therapy preserves both poles and oscillates between them.

Let me give an example: A patient talks about wanting to move from her large cluttered house to a small apartment furnished like those she had seen in Santa Fe: thick adobe walls, cool tile floors, an occasional Navajo rug, a few plants in unglazed pots, a skylight, a stone bench with cushions. This woman has spent her life in a traditional way, giving her time and energy to her husband and her three children. Now that her children have grown and moved out and her husband's career has been firmly established, she has begun tentatively to make a life for herself first as a volunteer and now as a paid administrator in an environmental protection organization.

Her fantasy is a metaphor for her striving for internal order and for a psychological space of her own that is not furnished with the accretions of other people's lives. The metaphor expresses the need to come into her own psychologically after years of turning outward toward others. She never does actually find or move into this dream apartment. But she does something else in the real world that becomes an approachable analogue. She converts one of her children's old bedrooms into a space for herself and she keeps it very sparse: a prayer rug, a single chair, a Jerusalem orange plant, a desk, and the few books she wants to read now. This move has happened because of an imperative from her unconscious for a compensating reversal. Jung has described this kind of "enantiodromia" (a reversal or turning into its opposite) as a common occurrence in midlife and beyond. The unconscious, in his view, attempts to correct for the imbalance of the first half of life. It is helpful for my patient and me to share the knowledge that the real and the metaphoric are interwoven, that rooms and houses have to do as well with bodies and psyches, that in remaking her space, as Yeats wrote of revising his poems, it was herself she remade. As she and I talked about these spaces, we shared an implicit knowledge that occasionally was made explicit: Sometimes she and I were talking about actual rooms, sometimes about inner space, and sometimes about both at the same time, inner and outer conjoined.

LITERALIZING OR "FREEZING" THEORETICAL METAPHORS

I have described the overzealous exploration of metaphor and the insufficient recognition of implicit metaphors as problems in therapeutic work. Now I want to address the way in which we as therapists can unwittingly be possessed by ruling metaphors of theory or metapsychology.

As long as we stay grounded in clinical experience we are generally aware of using metaphors ourselves or of a patient's explicit use of metaphors. In other words, we are aware that a lens is being used to look at reality, and that what we say depends to some extent on the lens as well as whatever is "out there." We are aware that we are making an approximation, creating a heuristic or a model. In these specific uses of metaphor, we recognize that the figures of speech are not statements about "reality" but are statements of our experience. Indeed, much therapeutic work consists of unfreezing the metaphors that have patients in their grip and of relativizing them, showing that their entrenched metaphors represent one way of looking at the world, but not necessarily the only way. In this aspect both we and our patients become aware that we are playing with a way of seeing.

But when we as therapists use large-scale theoretical metaphors unconsciously, then we run into trouble. This is what happens most often in the unspoken, implicit grand concepts we adopt about the nature and structure of the psyche or the analytic process. Used often and unquestioningly enough, any such explanatory construct begins to feel like the truth. When we reify "the unconscious" as a structure, an entity, rather than seeing the term as a shorthand noun to describe an attentional process—then *a* way of seeing becomes *the* way of seeing; instead of being a lens, it effectively serves as a set of blinders.

Of course, it is impossible to look at the world without a way of seeing; observation and attention can never be wholly objective and disinterested. The task is to become aware of our templates so we can realize what they let through and what they cover up.

A case in point is an article by Pederson-Krag (1956), which explicitly questions the too-literal use of large-scale metaphor in metapsychological theorizing. To think of the mind as a continent inhabited by warring nations is heuristically useful, she claims, but it does not explain anything. Pederson-Krag is hoist with her own petard, however, for the ubiquity of metaphor is inescapable. In her critique of the use of it in analytic thinking, she (Pederson-Krag, 1956) writes:

> when we try to delineate the psyche realistically, objectively, and without borrowed analogies, we find ourselves aligned with the physicists. For the ego is essentially a meeting place of forces, instinctual drives derived from the physiological needs

of the body on the one hand, and on the other, energies triggered by memories of the world without, superego and reality demands. (pp. 70–71)

It is striking that the author does not recognize that her description of the ego is *also* a metaphor (a meeting place of forces), and that literalizing that metaphor from kinetics will have its own set of consequences. The point is that we are inescapably drawn to make metaphoric models. In producing or in using theory, one must recognize that the map is not the territory, that these are "as-if" approximations.

A growing number of writers have decried operating out of frozen and unrecognized theoretical metaphors, among them Schafer (1976), Spence (1987), and Carveth (1984). Spence writes that metaphor is most useful when dealing with the unknown and the complex in a tentative way. And it is useful to the extent we are conscious of speaking or thinking in metaphors. Spence (1987) puts it as a paradox: "Their power as an aid to comprehension is directly proportional to our awareness of their metaphoric nature" (p. 4).

Problems arise when metaphors become reified or frozen or literalized. Spence cites the "archeological" metaphor used by Freud to describe analytic work and says that if this image is taken as an unquestioned given, rather than as a figure to be used deliberately and possibly rejected or modified, it has unfortunate unexamined consequences that really run counter to the nature of therapeutic experience. This metaphor of the archeologist/detective who "solves" the crime or reconstructs the artifact fosters the notion that there is a single solution to psychological puzzles (Spence, 1987):

> This axiom is deeply embedded in our psychoanalytic folklore; it assumes that there is a single meaning which is uppermost in any clinical fragment, that the context of the listener is irrelevant (because [the analyst's] personal needs and wishes can be set aside), and that the meaning of the protocol lies entirely "out there." (p. 57)

All this, says Spence, is entirely questionable. Indeed, it runs counter to Freud's frequently expressed view that every psychological event is multiply determined.

Another metaphor Spence seriously questions is that of the analyst's "freely hovering attention." This is a metaphor (attention is a suspended, vibrating neutral receiver) that has become literalized and taken as a shibboleth. When this happens, we are prevented from seeing its limitations as a truth-statement. Yes, of course it is possible at times to immerse oneself in a kind of reverie and listen to the "music" as well as the words of the therapeutic exchange without pushing for meaning or closure. But research on attention shows that almost all attention has some element of purpose and constructiveness. Therapists may differ in their ability or desire to release into reverie, but even those who choose to enter that state cannot and should not spend all their time there. In fact, as Carveth (1984) demonstrates, Freud himself did not adhere to the metaphor completely. "The analyst is a mirror," he says at one point, emphasizing the receptive, nonintrusive qualities of the therapist. And at another, "The analyst is a surgeon," emphasizing the active, intrusive behaviors of the analyst. Both of these are true—or better, both are suggestive of some aspect of the analytic attitude, and each rules out as well as illuminates some aspect of the therapeutic relationship.

Spence goes even farther than this. He wants us to become aware that "the unconscious" as a structural entity is itself a metaphor. He acknowledges that those of us who have assimilated the archeological view and the "reality" of the unconscious may be "shocked to be told that these are only figures of speech and that alternative metaphors are also available which might make even better sense of the clinical findings." He (Spence, 1987) goes on to acknowledge Freud's sensitivity to the issue, but adds that nevertheless, Freud sometimes blurred the distinction between "model and observation and tended to treat his metaphor as if it were a confirmed piece of reality. Many of his followers have made the same mistake" (p. 15). In the foreword to this book of Spence's, Jerome Bruner is even harsher:

> Psychoanalysis invoked positivism to legitimize its claim to being a deterministic science that dealt in causality, while at the same time robing its concepts in the metaphoric language of drama that effectively kept them from being testable, for metaphors have virtually no limit on their extension. (p. xi)

Classical Freudian metapsychology has no monopoly on such untestable metaphors. It has, perhaps, professed to be more scientific than other psychologies and hence is more open to question on those grounds. But "selfobjects," "internalized objects," "good and bad breasts," the "animus," the "shadow"—all these are metaphors. We cannot give them up, but we need to see each of them as one way of apprehending reality—not the only way. This perspective does not reduce metaphors to mere fancies or illusions. It acknowledges that metaphor is utterly central in apprehending the world. But only insofar as we are aware of metaphors *as* metaphors can we use them rather than being used *by* them. The more metaphor becomes established, the more likely we are to assume that that's how it is in the world. It takes on a self-fulfilling aspect. In Freud's defense, he did speak of metaphors as "scaffolding" around a structure, which presumably should not be confused with the structure itself (Freud, 1900). But in fact a number of Freudian metaphors have become foundations rather than scaffolds, and then they are hidden and no longer subject to revision or dismantling.

The most brilliant work I have seen on the coercive aspect of frozen metaphor is a paper by Carveth (1984), "The Analyst's Metaphors." He treats the subject in a number of ways, but the main pylon on which his discussion rests is the notion of "literalizing." As I see it, we literalize a metaphor when we literalize the figurative statement "A equals B." We treat that statement as a symbolic equation, an identity operation, an assertion that A intrinsically means B, rather than that this formulation is simply a way of speaking. When we *know* we are speaking metaphorically it is as if we are both inside and outside the statement of equality. We put quotations around the equals-sign so that the statement reads: A "equals" B. This is a *tentative* statement, emphasizing a similarity while at the same time recognizing it as only an approximation. This stance (A is and is really not B at the same time) is very close to what Winnicott talks about in transitional phenomena. Unless we can put quotes around the "equals" we are taking metaphor too literally and hence losing the advantage it can give us.

The conversion of metaphor into identity or essence ("A *intrinsically means* B") has clinical implications as well as theoretical ones. It puts us into what Carveth calls an "essentializing" mode rather than a "contextualizing" mode. Operating in the essentializing mode, one asks, "What is *the* meaning of a given statement or piece of behavior by the patient?" In the contextualizing mode, which represents depth psychology at its best, one asks, "What is the range of multiple, overdetermined meanings we can hypothesize for this statement or behavior?"

In clarifying this distinction, Carveth (1984) cites an illustration from Arlow's (1979) seminal paper on metaphor. In that paper, Arlow espouses a contextualizing position and criticizes Sharpe for the simple-mindedness of her "equations." According to Carveth, however, Arlow then goes on to give a case example that suffers from a similar reductionism: In this example, a woman patient complains to her student therapist about the sticky smelly stuff the beautician put on her hair; she wonders how the name "shrink" got applied to analysts; she muses about hostility she's been feeling toward men recently, talks about the house-painter who didn't put a sheet over the living room door while sandblasting, so that dirt spilled into the library; the air conditioning repairmen had come too late and the air conditioner had dripped condensed water on the floor, ruining the newly laid carpet. Arlow reports that the therapist asked the patient at that point, "Are you menstruating?" And she said "Yes. . . . I just began this morning. How did you know?" (p. 379).

The young analyst was intuitively correct, at one level, and he clearly stunned his patient with his intuition about her bodily functioning. But he seems to have been making the equation, "Messy liquid equals menstrual flow." As Carveth indicates, this is one "meaning" of the associations, and because it was "verified" it may seem to be the only meaning. But in fact, most analysts would want more of the patient's associations to her manifest statements. He (Carveth, 1984) writes:

> This material could be indicative of a woman's irritation at a man's premature ejaculations; a fear of pregnancy caused by his failure to take precautions; or even resentment at the analyst's "dirty" insinuations which sully and smear her character; among other possibilities. (p. 505)

"*Among other possibilities*"—that is the phrase that requires emphasizing. For when we "deliteralize" metaphors for ourselves and our patients by understanding that they are apt but partial, we gain flexibility and we model an openness to other possibilities. We may at times choose to sacrifice some flexibility—after all we cannot entertain all possibilities and see things from every point of view. But if we are conscious that other possible metaphors exist, we at least know that we are using our templates as templates.

In the next chapter, I will describe some of the large-scale templates that have been used to characterize the therapeutic process itself, metaphors of therapeutic interaction and of the therapeutic "space."

CHAPTER 8

Metaphors of the Therapeutic Encounter

To the extent that our "possession" by one or the other of this range of metaphors [of the analytic process] blinds us to other possible models, our work is to that degree rigid and we are to this same degree blind. Not only does the analyst's individual myth or "personal equation" influence his conception of the therapeutic process and his role as therapist, it also expresses itself in his most seemingly objective and scientific contributions.

—DONALD CARVETH, "The Analyst's Metaphors"

I n this chapter, we will look at a number of metaphors used to characterize either the therapeutic process or the therapeutic "space" in order to highlight their constructed nature. These metaphors are constructs and as such suitable for deconstruction and reconstruction, much as a patient's life history is a construction suitable to understanding and reworking.

Some of these metaphors of the therapeutic process—the frame, the container, the holding environment—have wide currency. Each has a special flavor reflecting in some ways the life experience or personal myth of the theorist. And each should have certain consequences for the therapeutic process that differentiate one from another.

FREUD AS A METAPHORIST OF THE THERAPEUTIC PROCESS

My own introduction to depth psychology was through reading the major works of the Freud canon. From the first, I was drawn to Freud

— 136 —

the writer as much as to Freud the metapsychologist. I experienced what Mahony (1982) has described so vividly in his *Freud as a Writer*: that is, Freud's enormous sense of his audience and the seeming immediacy and spontaneity that enable the reader to watch a great mind at work. This work often seems like play because of Freud's remarkable capacity to use figurative language to bring theory alive. (I think of the ego ridden by three masters, the likening of free association to the attentional process of a patient looking out the window of a moving train, the image of analysis as reclamation work, and so on.)

Because Freud was a master rhetorician, it is impossible to summarize his figures of speech in their richness and diversity, despite many attempts to do so (e.g., Trilling, 1940; Nash, 1962; Mahony, 1982; Shengold, 1981; Spence, 1987). His use of metaphoric analogies of enormous range makes his books as much works of art as attempts to construct a fledgling science. The vivacity of his style, indeed, won him the Goethe Prize for literature in 1935. Freud's metaphors cover the vast range of his erudition and are drawn from geology, chemistry, optics, hydraulics, and military strategy. Many of these metaphors were applied to his metapsychology, as heuristic devices. Freud (1900) himself was very aware of the limitations of metaphor, warning us in *The Interpretation of Dreams* (p. 536) that we "should not mistake the scaffolding for the building." Thus, he uses a metaphor to comment on the limitations of metaphor.

Although Freud was often highly interactive with his patients, his metaphors for the psychoanalytic process seem to reflect less a mutual impingement and engagement than (1) a parallel process, like two tracks running side by side, or (2) an interaction in which one of the participants (the analyst) does something to the other (the patient). In the first instance, the analyst's unconscious, accessed through free-floating attention, mirrors the patient's unconscious as it tries to speak through his halting and doomed attempts at free association. The analyst becomes the attuned spectator of the patient who, according to the fundamental rule enunciated at the outset, is to describe what goes through his head without censorship and without editing as though he were a passenger describing the scenery along the route of a moving train. The injunction is to "report everything you see," and the engagement comes as the unconscious of the analyst catches and reflects the unconscious of the patient.

The second kind of metaphor suggests a very asymmetrical relationship in which the analyst operates on or does something to the patient. (Freud says much less about how the patient operates on the analyst than do later writers who have paid more attention to counter-transference in all its cuing, interfering, and facilitating functions.) In his paper "Lines of Advance in Psychoanalytic Therapy," Freud (1919) writes that the psychology of the psychoanalytic process is so unique that it takes more than one analogy to represent it. He accordingly compares the work of the psychoanalyst to that of a chemist, surgeon, orthopedist, and teacher. This multiple comparison reflects Freud's respect for the complexity of psychic life and the consequent complexity of the work needed to explicate its mysteries.

Among Freud's most prominent metaphors for the process are those drawn from archeology. We know from the photographs of his consulting room how devoted he was to ancient artifacts—particularly Greek and Egyptian. And the idea of digging down into the earth for treasure suggests both the depth and the stratification of the psyche. In another famous metaphor, Freud (1933) writes of analytic work as reclamation work, "not unlike the draining of the Zuider Zee" (p. 80). These metaphors emphasize the arduous downward movement to the bedrock to get at what is original and primary in the psyche. But as I have noted, the idea of the analyst as archeological sleuth can have the unfortunate consequence of seeming to require a single solution. Another of Freud's recurring metaphors is of the analyst as surgeon, operating in a quasi-sterile field so as not to become contaminated with the *dreck* he is dealing with. The doctor must not be penetrated by the sepsis of the patient. Both the archeological and the surgical metaphors suggest "operations" of the analyst on a somewhat passive patient. The patient is either a layered structure that is being exposed or an immobilized surgical patient.

What do such metaphors entail? They *can* entail a situation of maximal psychological distance between analyst and patient, of maximal blankness of screen. Some followers of Freud, more royalist than the king, have made parodies of these metaphors. Just as Jung is reputed to have said, "Thank God I'm Jung and not a Jungian," Freud might have said, "Thank God I'm Freud and not a Freudian." For from what we know about his own practice Freud did many unorthodox, "unFreudian" things—extending hours, loaning money, occasionally making personal disclosures, and giving little lectures. But perhaps even more important, he did not appear to be the cool, impersonal psychological surgeon he was enjoining his followers to be. A number of accounts by his patients have corroborated the warmth of his engagement with them. Among the most feeling memoirs is that of Hilda Doolittle, the poet known as "H.D." (1984). She writes of the warm mutual appreciation she and Freud had for the artifacts in his consulting room, of his pleasure at her giving him flowers for his birthday. She also recounts his rueful response when she told him how maternal he was; patients kept saying this about him, he said, but he felt himself to be such a such a *masculine* man!

This side of Freud—his relatedness and warmth—emerges in his speaking and writing style as well. In giving lectures, according to Mahony (1982), Freud typically would fixate on a particular member of the audience he knew to be sympathetic to him and would address his remarks directly to him or her. (The "her" in many instances was his friend and follower, Lou Andreas-Salomé; in fact, in a letter to Lou, Freud wrote that her absence at his lecture had made him uncomfortable, as though he had lost an orientation point.) And in writing, he had an almost uncanny sense of the presence of the reader. Mahony tellingly points out that because he was not afraid to use the singular pronoun "I" in his writing, when he used "we," it did not seem to be the mechanical editorial "we" behind which scholarly writers hide themselves but rather a direct invitation to the reader to accompany him along the byways and turnings, cul-de-sacs, and royal roads to the unconscious. This vivid sense of his readers, leading him to cast his writing often in the form of real or imaginary lectures to an audience, could not have been divorced from his practice. Indeed, Mahony (1982) likens Freud's delivery of the *Introductory Lectures* over a two-year period to a gentle guiding and working through of his audience's resistance, as though the audience had become a kind of collective patient:

> We need only compare the beginning, when the very presence
> of psychoanalysis elicits audience resistance . . . to the end of
> the series the following year, when the meaning of symptoms
> and repression dawns upon the audience. . . . In sum, the text
> is a weaving of pedagogy and guided working through. (p. 95)

What are we to say, then, of this discrepancy between a number of the metaphors Freud used for the analytic process and his actual practice, which appears to have been more warm, humane, and flexible than his metaphors—geologist, chemist, surgeon, or even educator—might suggest? Perhaps we must invoke Freud's own caution about taking metaphors too literally. "The scaffolding is not the building." It may be that for personal–historic reasons, Freud's need to win acceptance from a scientific community still drenched with positivism and 19th-century mechanism led him to "force" his analogies, as a gardener "forces" flower growth. It may also be that Freud was still uneasy with his more feminine aspects, and that some of his own myth crept into his dictum in "Analysis Terminable and Interminable" (1937) that for men the great final task of psychoanalysis was to be able to value their feminine side. In any case this discomfort, including the discomfort at the maternal transference ("But I am such a *masculine* man!") may have unconsciously guided his use of metaphors that suggest complete objectivity, rigor, and exactness.

If one carried Freud's metaphors of the surgeon-practitioner or the archeologist-practitioner to their furthest points we would be seeing the following entailments:

1. A profound inequality in the relationship between analyst and patient. The analyst is the one who knows.
2. An attempt to guide at some point, even within the structure of free association.
3. A conception of the patient as someone acted on by the analyst's operations, be they cutting or digging. If the surgical model is pursued, does this mean that the patient is passive and anesthetized?
4. The heat of the interaction is not emphasized so much as the need for sober scrutiny and patient unearthing.

What emerges in this view I believe is a patriarchal model of a benign if distant father who "knows best." What it omits is the mutuality of affect and relationship and the perturbation in the joint field of the analyst and the patient. It entails a dichotomizing of psychological health and illness and a distance between patient and therapist in a "sterile field."

Yet, as I have said, we know in practice that Freud was more involved and more rule-breaking than these metaphors would suggest.

He did brief therapy on occasion (and all psychoanalysis was brief then by our standards—Freud felt called upon to warn his colleagues that psychoanalytic treatment might often extend up to a *year!*) He also lent a patient money; he offered reassurance. When H.D., who was six feet tall, commented on her excessive height, he told her his previous patient was even taller. He offered to lend her books. He accepted her gifts to him. And he created for this one highly creative patient, an atmosphere that was far different from the laboratory. The very profusion of artifacts in his consulting room—statues from Egypt, ancient Greece, and even an ivory Vishnu under a canopy of snake heads—made his office less a physician's consulting room and more a museum or even a temple. H.D. recounts a dream that took place in a cathedral. Of it she said, "It is really the Cathedral that is all important. Inside the Cathedral we find regeneration and reintegration. This room [Freud's office] is the Cathedral."

What are we to make of this testimony? Is this merely the idealizing transference of a brilliant and highly spiritual patient? Or was Freud's practice far more complex and flexible than his metaphors could allow because of the intellectual climate of the time, his need to gain legitimacy, and his internal struggles about feeling? It seems as though his metaphors of the impersonal, uninvolved practitioner have been taken literally by anxious analytic candidates and by generations of followers who are compelled to make their science ever more stringent. These metaphors may have been created for acceptability from the community, but Freud was able to break his own rules because he was a creator, not a follower, and because the rules had not yet been engraved in stone.

JUNG'S PSYCHOTHERAPEUTIC SPACE AS *TEMENOS,* CIRCLE, AND VESSEL

I now turn to work of the other great pioneer of depth psychology, C. G. Jung, in order to make some inferences about his view of the psychotherapeutic space. I say "inferences" because only in his "Psychology of the Transference" (Jung, 1946) did he make explicit the analogy between what happens in the analytic process and what the alchemists were attempting in their work of transforming base matter into the precious "lapis" or living philosopher's stone. Jung believed that the medieval alchemists were protopsychologists who were using the only language and symbols available to them to talk about the transformation of unconsciousness into consciousness and about finding the center of the personality, which Jung has termed the Self, or the archetype of wholeness. In this psychological drama, Jung draws on plates of an alchemical text, the *Rosarium Philosophorum*, to depict a process in which the adept and his *soror* (sister)—like therapist and patient—together go about the "opus" or work of transformation that involves various stages of blackening, putrefaction, union in a bath, dismemberment, and production finally of a hermaphroditic child that embodies the opposites.

This union or *coniunctio* of adept and soror, parallels the conjunction of the analyst and patient in the course of therapeutic work, and serves as an interpersonal representation of what is inevitably an intrapsychic process: The patient becomes conjoined with the disowned or unconscious aspects of himself to become both more individuated and more able to contain in consciousness the opposites that he or she embodies.

The three key metaphors that are related to this process of integration are the *temenos* (the sacred precinct), the vessel, and the circle, and they intertwine in the writing of Jung. Perhaps the most advanced graphic representations of these forms are to be found in the mandalas that occur in Tibetan religious art. But Jung observed that people the world over draw circles as symbols of wholeness and that patients in producing drawings in the course of analysis often spontaneously draw recurring forms of squares embedded in circles.

The Greek word *temenos* (Jung, 1952) refers to a sacred precinct, a piece of land, such as a grove, that has been set apart and dedicated to a god, as the precinct of Olympia was dedicated to the earth goddess Gaia. This sacred space could be a castle, a city, or courtyard; it could be quadratic or circular. Its sacredness was assured by having priests designate a boundary around it—a charmed or protective circle. This magic circle has very ancient origins; originally it was a furrow drawn around a sacred precinct or temple to guard against distracting or profane influences from the outside and to protect the contents from escaping. Thus, priests of old would circumambulate a city to demarcate its limits and offer prayers of protection, just as someone digging for treasure would draw a circle around a field to keep away evil. In the Christian era, the idea of the *temenos* was expanded to include cloisters and walled secluded gardens, which were often associated in Christian iconography with the Virgin Mary.

Jung (1929) makes the analogy to the psychological domain when he speaks of a circle drawn around the sacred temple "of the innermost personality in order to prevent an 'outflowing' or to guard by apotropaic [i.e., warding off] means against distracting influences from outside." In another instance, Jung (1944) describes a patient's dream of a snake making a circle around the dreamer who remains "rooted to the ground like a tree" as describing both the magic circle and what it demarcates—the *temenos*: "a taboo area where he will be able to meet the unconscious" (p. 54).

This area in the psyche, I believe, can easily be objectified in the external world in an arena that is dedicated specifically to meeting the unconscious—namely, the therapeutic space. In this *temenos*, or "taboo" area, what is inside does not leak out and what is outside does not break in. It is set off from the ordinary world by a magic circle of privacy, quiet, closed doors, and fixed time—as well as by the protective steadiness of the therapist.

Jung sometimes emphasizes the "sacred" or "taboo" area of the *temenos* itself and sometimes the magic circle that bounds it; occasionally he changes the metaphor to talk of a vessel or container for psychic contents. In the lectures he gave (in English) to an audience at Tavistock in 1935, Jung was asked to diagnose and comment on two drawings made by a patient of one of the psychoanalysts in the audience. They were drawings of figured vases. The first was enormously lopsided and tilted, with peculiar lines dividing the field, suggesting a major skewing of the psyche of this patient, whom Jung correctly intuited to be schizophrenic. The second drawing, made after some period of therapeutic work, was much more ordered: The vase stood on its base and was altogether more "legible." Jung (1935) comments, "The idea of a receptacle is an archetypal idea . . . It is the idea of a magic circle which is drawn round something that has to be prevented from escaping or protected against hostile influences" (p. 178).

The containing vessel in which the work of transformation occurs is seen most clearly in the alchemical text and pictures from which Jung (1946) draws analogies for the psychotherapeutic process.

The transformation of base matter into a higher form requires a well-sealed vessel (*vas bene clausum*) to withstand the heat of the transformative process. In describing the alchemical furnace, Jung talks of a vessel that is hermetically sealed, that is round or egg-shaped; this becomes the "matrix" or uterus from which the wondrous philosopher's stone would be born. In some of the alchemical texts, the practitioner and his sister are in a bath together (i.e., they are in the unconscious together in the therapeutic vessel). In others, where the furnace analogy is used, the dangerous heat of the process is emphasized. In pointedly relating alchemical and analytic work, Jung (1946) says specifically: "Alchemy describes, not merely in general outline but often in the most astonishing detail, the same psychological phenomenology which can be observed in the analysis of unconscious processes" (p. 198).

Jung (1946) portrays how harrowing these processes can be, as the ego becomes tossed about, consciousness is temporarily unseated, and a terror overwhelms the patient:

> It is like passing through the valley of the shadow, and sometimes the patient has to cling to the doctor as the last remaining shred of reality. This situation is difficult and distressing for both parties; often the doctor is in much the same position as the alchemist who no longer knew whether he was melting the mysterious amalgam in the crucible or whether he was the salamander glowing in the fire. Psychological induction inevitably causes the two parties to get involved in the transformation of the third and to be themselves transformed in the process, and all the time, the doctor's knowledge, like a flickering lamp, is the one dim light in the darkness. (pp. 198–199)

The alchemical texts also tell us, according to Jung (1955), that the circle and vessel are the same—the mandala seen in the dreams and drawing of patients is indeed the "vessel of transformation" (p. 16). The therapeutic situation becomes a replica of the internal situation, and what starts out as an interpersonal process (the *coniunctio* between patient and therapist) is itself a metaphor for and a step toward an internal integration between conscious and hitherto unconscious aspects of the patient's psyche.

What are the entailments of Jung's view of the psychotherapeutic space as a *temenos* surrounded by a magic circle or as a vessel in which contents are held under pressure and transformed by the heat? I believe that Jung affirms the importance of the well-sealed, well-bounded space as an essential protection for the difficult work of accessing and transforming unconscious impulses, fantasies, images. He also insists that the space so demarcated or the vessel so sealed is the area of *symbolic* interactions. But two themes are qualitatively unique in his metaphors of the circle, the *temenos* precinct, and the vessel: One is the heat of the encounter within that space, and the other is its sacred or numinous quality.

First, the heat. It is so intense that it can illuminate and scorch both participants; indeed, Jung holds that the analyst in an intensive engagement is also changed by the process. This is a far cry from the metaphor of the analyst-surgeon or the analyst-archeologist, someone who operates on or unearths, protected by his expertise and self-scrutiny. What Jung describes are moments of uncertainty, terror, and sometimes of a *participation mystique,* in which both participants are in the vessel or in the bath together—confused, frightened, and having as their only protection against disintegration the frail and sometimes flickering light of the therapist's reason. Occasionally, in Jung's own experience, that light was snuffed out. The transference, which at times seemed to him like "the alpha and omega" of the analytic process, at others seemed just a painful burden. Carotenuto (1982) and Goodheart (1984) have given examples of Jung's countertransference being unacknowledged, especially in his early work.

Second, the sacred. Perhaps because of such experiences of the archetypal power of the *coniunctio* or union, the analytic space is represented by Jung as the home of the *numen,* a divine—if sometimes demonic—presiding spirit. Not only is it an area of taboo that has a taken on a quasi-religious force. It is also the arena in which a kind of sacred marriage takes place—first between patient and analyst, ultimately between the patient's ego and the deeply unconscious contrasexual animus or anima. The "something more" that is transacted in this *temenos* is not just the symbolic. It is the push toward realization of the Self. The capital-S "Self" in the Jungian view is the archetype of order and wholeness; when it manifests we recognize it with wonder and with awe. Such was the experience of my patient Sylvia, who for the first time moved out of a confining relationship to be on her own: Her dream image of walking through a tunnel of light, surrounded and imperceptibly contained by its nacreous glow, reflected the ecstasy that such manifestations evoke.

— 145 —

LANGS AND MILNER: TWO VIEWS OF THE THERAPEUTIC FRAME

A number of writers have referred to the therapeutic/analytic encounter as taking place within a frame. I should like to single out two of them—Robert Langs and Marion Milner—to show how a similar metaphor can take on a very different feeling tone in the hands of two practitioners who differ profoundly in psychological style.

Langs's Use of the Frame

Robert Langs is probably the most vigorous, consistent, and insistent spokesman for attending to the frame in work with patients. Langs is often persuasive, and his reminders of the negative consequences of ubiquitous inattention to frame issues are extremely useful. Yet I see in him an arrogance posing as openness, a substitution of "blaming the resident" (much of his work consists of seminar notes of work with young residents) for "blaming the patient." He comes across as a gigantic Logos figure, a superego of the Word who constantly says, "Thou shalt not." Despite his protests that his point of view is not mechanical, inhumane, or uncaring, one need only read these transcripts to see how his commitment to "the Truth" overrides his concern for his students and *their* vulnerability.

In addition to the listening process, Langs (1978) puts the frame (alternatively referred to as the framework or the ground rules) at the center of his therapeutic system. In his most explicit and extended treatment of the frame—*The Therapeutic Environment* (1979)—Langs defines the frame as the ground rules that create a "basic hold" for therapist and patient and that differ from conditions outside the frame. He also distinguishes between the "fixed frame" and the "variable frame." The fixed frame includes complete confidentiality, absence of any third party involvement (including insurance companies), fixed number of sessions per week, patient's physical orientation (face-to-face or on couch), fee (unchanged throughout the course of the therapy and charged for every hour for which the therapist is present), full attention of the therapist during the hour without interruptions by telephone, etc. For Langs, these are the sine qua non of a therapeutic holding environment, and they should not be modified; if they are modified, the damage must be detected and the frame "rectified" as quickly as possible. The variable frame, which is by its nature more subject to slight human variation, has to do with the anonymity and the neutrality of the therapist and the nature of his or her interpretations.

Langs rightly says that for teaching purposes, one learns more when things go awry. But unfortunately, in the clinic setting in which his residents have worked, by its very nature things go awry almost all the time: Intrusive third parties (secretaries, receptionists who collect bills, etc.) are ubiquitous, group intakes are held before the patient sees his or her therapist, offices may have to be changed, and the training status of the therapist and the artificial termination of therapy are all special constraints. These offer plenty of opportunities to discuss the importance of maintaining the frame and the costs of breaking it. Langs's idea that alterations in the frame evoke strong unconscious emotional reactions and serve as major "adaptive contexts" around which derivative associations will accrue seems to me to be a useful and demonstrable principle. It is important to be attentive to the underlying threat expressed in derivatives to the overt gratitude a patient may express for a therapist's violating the frame by extending the hour, rescheduling, etc. Such changes in the frame may, indeed, be accompanied by associations that present themes of assault, danger, and invasion or seduction. (I gave such an example in Chapter 7.) And they may be accompanied by actions through which patients attempt to underline for the therapist the need to rectify the frame: missing the rescheduled hour, coming late after a therapist has rescheduled a previous hour, and so on.

Langs's (1979) warning that the patient will feel threatened by such concessions is an important directive and corrective to therapists. He states this warning, however, not as a possibility but as a certainty: Any such "gratification" must be perceived by patients as a confession that the therapist cannot manage his or her inner mental state and therefore is not a safe container for the patient's projective identifications. This is a hypothesis that Langs never fails to confirm.

Furthermore, Langs asserts unequivocally that variations in the frame are the way the therapist acts out his or her unresolved countertransferences and that *all* deviations in the frame have the effect of infantilizing the patient. I do not agree. Raising a patient's fee, for example, may give him or her a message of the expectation of competence, which is quite the opposite of infantilization. Moreover, again looking at Langs's style and rhetoric, it is the relentlessness with which this idea is pursued and the messianic rhetoric surrounding it that give one pause. Langs (1979) tells us that some therapists regard ground-rule departures as relatively insignificant, but "We are here to discover the truth of the matter" (p. 49). His hectoring tone cannot be accounted for solely by these departures. It is of a piece with his talk about "lie therapy" versus "truth therapy." To talk about "the Truth" strikes me as doctrinal and hence anti-scientific.

Langs avers in *The Therapeutic Environment* that, while his ground rules may seem excessively stringent, in fact, their very essence in the therapeutic experience is intensely human and rich in conscious and, especially, unconscious communication. He insists that the frame per se or the frame as an isolated set of rules means nothing but only signifies as a communication from the therapist to the patient. He (Langs, 1979) also writes:

> Do not allow the framework analogy to suggest something wooden, inanimate, nonhuman or isolated. The therapeutic framework is a very human frame filled with fluctuating unconscious communications. It is a way of holding the patient, offering him a sense of safety, creating conditions for open communication. (p. 108)

And yet I am left with the sense that something inhumane is going on here, that the therapist functions as a scientist/hypothesis tester engaged in the purely cognitive activity of searching for clues. Langs talks with approval of Bion's notion of the therapist approaching each hour without memory and without desire, and of engaging in a kind of reverie. "Reverie" suggests a dreamy free-floating attention that is neither passive nor active but is receptive; it is the state that Winnicott maintains is necessary between mother and infant. Langs's idea of "reverie" runs counter to the etymology of the word (*rêve* = dream) and to every association most people would bring to it. How a therapist constantly ferreting out the adaptive context, framing silent hypotheses, and checking them out can be in a state of reverie is incomprehensible to me. The analogy is more to a running computer than to a dreamy listener. Moreover, implied in Langs's system is the view that only the therapist's cognitive responses count—his (I say

— 148 —

"his" because Langs's bias is almost always to say "his") hunches, gut feelings, and affects are not emphasized as sources of information. Again, the rhetoric is revealing: A "hypothesis" has an entirely different associative net from a "hunch." Langs pays lip service to the play space that is created when the frame is secure. But there is so little evidence of any kind of play or reverie in Langs's instructional style that one wonders how it would find its way into work with patients. Langs himself would undoubtedly point out that the adaptive context of teaching is different from that of doing therapy. Nevertheless, "the style is the man," and the disclaimers about the humaneness of the frame do not ring true when we attend to the *music*—rather than merely the words—of Langs's discourse.

Despite the usefulness of becoming aware of the importance to the patient of even seemingly small variations, Langs's frame often feels to me like a Procrustean bed. It appears to be made of a hard, inflexible material, like heavy metal, that does not accommodate occasional bending or stretching. What's more, the frame does not demarcate or set off a picture, it becomes more important than the picture. The idea that frames might be slightly different for different patients is apparently anathema to Langs. When a resident suggested that perhaps a frame could be introduced that departed from Langs's specifications in some major respect but was consistently maintained, Langs replied that the frame he outlines with all dimensions fixed as he has described them has been shown to work best. There *is* something mechanical and doctrinaire about treating every patient in exactly the same way; all that varies, presumably, is the nature of the interpretations, and an occasional concession with depressed patients that the therapist be a little less silent than with others.

My own metaphorical speculation is that frames should be steady and secure, but perhaps they can be made of a material that is somewhat elastic and resilient, that conforms in some way to the shape of what is being framed. To pursue the analogy, one type of material cannot be used to frame every painting. Some look best in plexiglass, where the frame is virtually invisible; some require heavy gilded wood; others look best when contained and outlined in thin metal. When a painting is framed, the frame is not negligible. If the frame were to break, the painting might fall and be destroyed. But just as the scaffold is not the building, so the frame is not the painting.

Milner's Use of the Frame Metaphor

I want to contrast Langs's use of the frame with the view of the frame and understanding of the psychoanalytic process developed by Marion Milner, a British psychoanalyst perhaps insufficiently known to American psychotherapists. Milner is the author of half a dozen books—one of which, *The Suppressed Madness of Sane Men* (1987), is a collection of her seminal articles having to do with the symbolizing process in psychoanalysis and in art. *The Hands of the Living God* (Milner, 1969) is the account of the analysis of a schizophrenic woman through her drawings. *On Not Being Able to Paint* (Milner, 1957) explores the unconscious blocks to the creative process based on the author's own experience as an amateur painter. *A Life of One's Own*, her earliest book—published in 1935 under a pseudonym (Joanna Field) and reissued in 1981—attempts to account empirically for what gives her happiness and pleasure. This pursuit takes her on a journey through the labyrinth of thought, attention, dream, and consciousness. Something of her style can be seen from the chapter summary of her retrospective chapter:

> I had discovered something about happiness
> And found that science could help me, but was not the end
>   of my journey   -
> I thought I had discovered the critical point of willing
> And when I did what I could, then I became aware of an un-
>   conscious wisdom that was wiser than I. (p. ix)

The process by which she arrived at that wisdom was to use a kind of automatic writing (very like free associating or true reverie) to tap into what the unconscious was saying. She (Field [Milner], 1981) also learned to pay attention to bodily cues:

> Experiencing the present with the whole of my body instead of with the pinpoint of my intellect led to all sorts of new knowledge and new contentment. I began to guess what it might mean to live from the heart instead of the head, and I began to feel movements of the heart which told me more surely what I wanted than any making of lists. (pp. 176–177)

With remarkable awareness of her own process, she speaks of attention as a rhythm, oscillating between focus and drifting: It was the drifting that allowed the preconscious to speak and that permitted her to catch what she calls "butterflies," the merest flutterings of thought, affect, and bodily sensation that often led to real insight. She argues against any onesided truth and plumps for the need for both purposefulness and dreaminess, consciousness and surrender—a "female" receptivity and a "male" active watching and sifting. She speaks of true reflectivity in almost Jungian terms, though she was not a Jungian, as a means of allowing the internal male and female to interact. "Surely," she writes (Field [Milner], 1981), "the wide knowing is a containing act, as against a male penetrating one" (p. 225).

I include this quotation because this spirit informs Milner's second book as well. *An Experiment in Leisure* (published originally in 1937 and reissued in 1987) is a brilliant evocation of introverted intuition and the power of subjective nonlinear thinking. This intuitive curiosity and resonance to the symbolic also inform Milner's later psychoanalytic writing. These beliefs, originally applied to her own inner rhythms, became translated to her work as an analyst. They allowed her a freedom to move between action and contemplation, cognition and reverie, conscious and unconscious. It is an oscillation that operates also in the work of Milner's colleague, D. W. Winnicott, a man with an unusually well-developed feminine aspect.

The differences in temperament and style between Milner and Langs are reflected in the way Milner writes about the frame. She writes exploratorily, with a sense of wonder, and with the emphasis where it rightly should be—on the thing that is framed, not on the frame itself. She puts the analytic process in the wider context in which it belongs, the context of human symbolizing activity. In her words (Milner, 1957):

> Frames can be thought of both in time as well as in space and in other human activities beside painting. An acted play is usually, nowadays, framed by the stage, in space, and by the raising and lowering of the curtain in time. Rituals and processions are usually framed in space by barriers or by the policemen that keep back the onlookers. Dreams are framed in sleep and the material of a psychoanalytic session is framed both in space and time. And paintings, nowadays, are usually bounded by frames . . . Thus when there is a frame it surely serves to indicate that what's inside the frame has to be interpreted in a different way

> from what's outside it. . . . . Thus the frame marks off an area within which what is perceived has to be taken symbolically, while what is outside the frame is taken literally. Symbolic of what? We certainly assume that it is symbolic of the feelings and ideas of whoever determined the pattern or form within the frame. We assume that it makes sense, for instance we assume that the people on the stage are not there just by accident. In the same way, as analysts, we have learnt by experience that an apparently casual remark made within the frame of the session also makes sense if understood symbolically. (pp. 157–158)

Milner thus comes close to the Winnicottian view of potential or transitional space, where something is itself and not-itself at the same time: In therapy, a casual remark is a casual remark and has a heavily fraught subtext; the therapist is the therapist and also the patient's father, brother, mother, lover, etc. She puts the frame where it belongs: It is not a pillory, a procrustean bed, or even a rigid boundary demarcation but a heuristic. The frame is there to mark the entryway to the symbolic. Whenever we see or experience a frame, we are subliminally given the message, "Welcome to symbol land." The emphasis is on what is in the frame rather than the frame itself. This certainly makes sense. In most situations the frame should be barely visible, inviting one to suspend disbelief and enter into the framed area in the spirit of "as if." In a part of the passage above that I omitted, Milner writes that wall paintings that are not framed and paintings on the walls of caves (as in the great caves of Lascaux) come to resemble dream images—precisely *because* they are not framed. Instead, they blend into their surroundings and even draw on the topographic features of the walls themselves: a hole in the cave wall, for instance, has become an eye in the painting. Painters nowadays, not so interested in creating a nearly hallucinatory image, frame their works. But I think of the famous painting by René Magritte in which a line indicating the border of the canvas is set around a painting of the painter's studio, so that the painting and the surrounding room blend into each other, teasing us with the question of where does one begin and the other leave off?

In therapy, the frame must be secure enough to hold the symbolic activity but unobtrusive enough to allow the space for the transitional properties of the therapeutic encounter to occur. For me,

Langs's frame obtrudes to the point of dominating the picture. I am reminded of my dream about my patient in which the obvious absurdity of the dictum "The egg should fit the egg-cup" became clear. No, the egg-cup should fit the egg. And it may be, Langs to the contrary notwithstanding, that different patients need frames that are made of different metaphoric materials, and that when the frame is most easily and securely maintained, one is scarcely aware of it at all. It becomes like the edge of the Magritte canvas: an almost nonexistent line separating the real from the symbolic or imaginal. Indeed, perhaps the most important events in a therapy occur at the interface of the real/not-real, the area of illusion. This brings me to Winnicott's metaphor of "potential space."

WINNICOTT'S HOLDING ENVIRONMENT
AND POTENTIAL SPACE

I have said that the choice of metaphors is both reflective and determinative: The therapist's "personal myth" shapes the metaphors he or she will use, and these in turn, become filters through which experience is passed.

D. W. Winnicott, beginning as a pediatrician, had ample opportunity to see mothers and babies. His formulations about mothering (maternal preoccupation, the "good-enough mother," the facilitating or holding environment, which is ordinarily constant and free from gross psychological desertions or impingements) describe the conditions for healthy infant development (Winnicott, 1958). They also describe the psychoanalytic process, particularly when patients regress to near-infantile states and are unconsciously seeking to redo the mother–infant relationship in a safe and containing space.

Winnicott's (1971) emphasis is on the hold based neither on rules nor on structure but on the analyst as a containing presence. Clearly, he could depart from rules when necessary—regularly serving tea and biscuits to one severely deprived woman, making sure another patient waited in his waiting room until she had collected herself sufficiently after a session to be able to face the world, and so on. The hold comes from a therapist who can tighten or loosen the grasp in intuitive accord with particular patients, just as good-enough mothers do with their babies. If the grasp is too loose, the baby (the patient) will feel unprotected and in danger of falling; if it is too tight, the baby (patient) will feel constricted and pinioned. The maternal arms are human arms, firm but made of flesh rather than of wood, metal, or stone, and her framing arms are responsive to the needs of her particular child.

As important as the hold is the symbolic space in which the patient and analyst/mother engage. In talking of infant development, Winnicott (1971) introduced the by now widely known notion of transitional phenomena. Transitional objects are the first material objects that are both surrogates for the mother and extensions of self, existing midway between inner and outer, baby and mother, real and illusionary. Winnicott has described the paradox of these blankets, stuffed animals, pillows (what the small son of a friend of mine once described as "my loving thing") that are both invented and discovered by the infant. The baby must be allowed to preserve the paradox that the magic blanket existed all along out there, waiting to be discovered, and conversely that he or she created it. This transitional object is the first symbol, the first mediator between the baby's needs and the outer world, the first thing that "stands for." And it is in this realm of transitional space, of "creative illusion," that all play, art, and eventually culture develop.

Winnicott makes two major contributions in this regard. First, in emphasizing the reenactment of mother/infant interchange in the analytic process he gives analysis a very different cast from the cognitive, interpretive, logos-oriented patriarchal cast of classical psychoanalysis. The reexperiencing and reworking of a process takes precedence over the authoritative Word.

Second, what makes Winnicott's work analytic is his steadfast emphasis on the symbolic. The holding environment creates a particular metaphorical kind of space. He refers to it variously as transitional space, the play space, or potential space. In this space the wounds of early mismatches or traumata can be healed, and the symbol-making capacity enhanced or restored.

Let me give an example: Although Winnicott did feel free at times to depart from neutrality and even from the traditional taboo against touching patients, his more characteristic stance is indicated in the following interchange with an adult male patient he described in *Fragment of an Analysis*, published in a posthumous volume of his essays (1987). The patient had expressed the wish that Winnicott would hold him, and Winnicott replied that if he did hold him, the patient would be aware of the awkwardness of the situation: one grown man holding another. Indeed, the literalness of the encounter would blot out the infantile experience that the patient was reliving. What was required was a symbolic holding. And that was provided by the couch. The patient was finally able to say to Winnicott, "*You* are the couch." The couch had become a transitional object, and the patient was able to see that such objects can "stand for" something else in a less encumbering way.

This patient could also experience himself as composite: He both was and was not the infant yearning for the maternal embrace; he both was and was not the adult who could understand the need to keep the holding metaphorical rather than actual.

The space existing between therapist and patient has become increasingly emphasized in the British "middle-school" of object relations (Winnicott, Balint, Fairbairn, Guntrip, Milner, Khan). This holding environment in some ways parallels the good-enough maternal environment, but it is not consciously aimed at reparenting or providing a corrective emotional experience (although it undoubtedly does some of these things). Creating such an environment is not an attempt to produce specific effects but rather to set up an atmosphere, climate, or space in which psychological change can occur. The analogy is to a physical space that is uncluttered, quiet, private, yet not cold or sterile, that does not impinge in startling ways, as photographs of a therapist's family would impinge in the consulting room. This space need not be bland or totally anonymous, just as the therapist need not be bland or totally anonymous. Such a physical environment—protected, quiet, warm, and responsive—is the physical analogue of a similar psychological space.

In this protected/protecting space, a kind of benign illusion or "as if" takes place: Two can become one, the new becomes the old, and, just as important, the old becomes new. In this space, distinctions between me and not-me, real and not-real, here and not-here, now and not-now blur and shift. This is the symbolic space. It is the area of imaginative play in which the most potent metaphor in all of psychotherapeutic work—the transference—is allowed to flourish and develop.

"Metaphor" and "transference" in fact bear the same etymological stamp. (*Metaphorein* in Greek means to carry over; *transferre* in Latin means to bear across). The therapist is both a real person, him- or herself—"my therapist"—*and* at the same time "my mother/father/ husband/wife/lover/brother/sister/son/daughter." And in this space of illusion, the projections or projective identifications are allowed and held until the patient can realize that the therapist is *not* his alcoholic father, her depressed mother, his hated sibling, or her magic savior.

Winnicott's "system" is less a system than a collection of resonant images and metaphors. Most assuredly an intuitive type in Jungian typological terms, Winnicott did not develop axioms or postulates; his thought seems to leap from intuition to intuition. A recent explication by Ogden (1986) has clarified and systematized Winnicott's complex notion of potential space. I have reviewed Ogden's summary in some detail elsewhere (Siegelman, 1989). I will briefly recapitulate it here.

Ogden tells us that this very embracing concept of Winnicott's includes the play space, the area of transitional phenomena, the analytic space, and the area of cultural experience and creativity. The notion of potential space has been enigmatic because it has been cast in a web of metaphoric images.

Ogden (1986) attempts to systematize Winnicott's main points as follows: Potential space originates in a physical and mental space that is potentially present between mother and infant. Later the infant can develop its own capacity to create this space. The implication is that the space must first exist between mother and infant in order for the infant to develop it on his or her own. There are two conditions in which the infant cannot generate this illusionary space: (1) when there is only fusion between mother and developing infant, with no possibility of separation or (2) when there is only separation with no illusion of merger. (I shall have more to say about these deformations of the symbol-making capacity in the next chapter.)

Winnicott (1971) has written, "Potential space . . . is the hypothetical area that exists (but cannot exist) between the baby and the object (mother or part of mother) during the phase of the repudiation of the object as not-me, that is, at the end of being merged in with the object" (p. 107). The formulation "that exists (but cannot exist)" embodies precisely the kind of paradox that Winnicott loves so dearly and that sums up a logical contradiction that is nevertheless a psychological truth. Something cannot be A and not-A at the same time—or so the logicians tell us. And yet that is *precisely* what a metaphor is, and what a symbol is: something that is itself and not itself at the same time.

In Winnicott's view, these paradoxes and contradictions *must* be maintained. Thus, the question "Did you find that [the transitional object] or did you invent it?" is never put to the infant. He or she must be able to believe both that the object was his own creation and that it already existed for him to find. As the space between infant and mother threatens to increase, it becomes filled in with this kind of symbolic illusion that turns the space into the realm of creative play. This space is an intermediate area that lies between inner psychological reality and external reality—"between the subjective object and the object objectively perceived, between me-extensions and what is not-me" (Winnicott, 1971, p. 100).

The transference is a similarly perfect ground for creating and later revising the view of the therapist as the patient's me-extension. The mother–infant situation is replayed and reworked in the therapeutic/analytic interchange. Both evoke the paradoxes of separateness in unity, of oneness in twoness, of twoness in oneness (the ability to be alone in the presence of the mother). The process represents a delicate oscillation between "we are one" and "we are two"—and sometimes the illusion that both are true simultaneously.

Ogden tells us that unity does not require and cannot produce symbols. Duality does. The psychological differentiation of mother and infant as objects, leads to a "third thing," the infant as subject, the creator of symbols. When the infant as subject becomes aware of his or her subjectivity, not only symbol-making becomes possible but also the beginning of concern for the other—of empathy, guilt, mourning, and reparation. Melanie Klein's "depressive position," like Winnicott's "position of concern" depends on the capacity to form symbols.

Empathy thus occurs within potential space, within the dialectic of being and not being the other. It is neither sustained merger nor utter separateness but an oscillation between merger and separation. The knowledge of the potential space prevents getting trapped in the Other. The knowledge of the actual or symbolic connection prevents being cut off from the Other.

Just as this dialectic is modeled for infants by mothers, so, I believe, is it also modeled for patients by therapists. The therapist's ability to oscillate between identification and separateness in which the patient is experienced alternately as subjective object and objective object—this serves as an implicit model for the patient. The patient is aware at some preconscious nonverbal level of the oscillations in the self and the other that sustain the illusion of potential space. These oscillations also make possible the kind of play that occurs in a developing therapy (Ogden, 1986), characterized by "humor, surprise, discovery, or originality" (p. 230).

My own intuition is that a spatial metaphor cannot ultimately describe a depth therapy or analysis. Within the space something happens. That something is the kind of oscillation I have been talking about, what Winnicott calls a "to-ing and fro-ing." The oscillation is not just an interpersonal process between therapist and patient but an internal process in each of them. The therapist oscillates between different levels of awareness and participation, from temporary mergers or identifications to a more rational stepping back and reflecting, from states of reverie to moments of clarity, from image to word.

One hopes that eventually this kind of oscillation becomes possible for the patient, too, so that he or she is not stuck for long periods in monolithic feeling states of depression or regression or caught in an intractable view of the world or of the therapeutic process. Perhaps the most useful thing the therapist models for the patient is this psychological suppleness: the ability to shift attention and levels of consciousness, to range up and down, in and out, back and forth. This flexibility may be communicated at totally subliminal levels. But it seems to me to call for a different analogy from any we have seen so far. The analogy is to the arts that move in time, and that move us as they move, to music and dance. I will return to this metaphor of the therapeutic process at the end of the next chapter.

CHAPTER 9

The Symbolic Attitude

*. . . images that are true symbols . . . are the best possible
expressions for something unknown—bridges thrown out towards an
unseen shore.*

C. G. JUNG, "On the Relation of Analytical Psychology to Poetry"

I n this chapter, I want to open metaphor outward, to show
that it is one aspect of the symbolic imagination in poets and
patients and of the symbolic attitude we take toward our work as
therapists. Imagination is a word with a long history, exalted by
Wordsworth and the Romantic poets, but often pathologized by be-
haviorists on one side and by some classical Freudians on the other. In
my reading of bridge figures like Rycroft and the British middle-school
of object relations theorists, I detect a growing wish to value and
redeem the imagination.

JUNG'S VIEW OF THE SYMBOLIC

Jung never had any doubt about the value of the imagination. As far
back as 1916, he was developing the idea of a "transcendent function"—transcendent used in a descriptive, not a mystical or evalua-
tive, way. This was simply that "third thing" that transcends two
domains when there is a dialogue between them. He envisaged this
happening in "active imagination"—a process by which a person
loosens his conscious focus, puts him- or herself in a state of reverie,
and allows psychological contents, such as a dream image, to emerge
and to become elaborated. This embellished product of the uncon-

scious then becomes a partner in a dialogue with the patient's ego in which neither dominates. What results is a symbolic product (using the written word or paint or clay) that contains elements of both. There is a foreshadowing here of what Kris (1952) was later to call "regression in the service of the ego," expressing the notion that temporary regression could lead to better integration. But perhaps Jung would have characterized the process as oscillation in the service of the Self. The notion of a mediating third thing that bridges domains through imagination also anticipates Winnicott's work on transitional objects and transitional phenomena.

Furthermore, Jung insisted on the distinction between a symbol and a sign. A sign is arrived at by convention and agreement; there is no necessary connection between it and what it denotes. There is no essential reason why a blinking yellow light should mean "slow down" except that we have chosen to make it mean that. A sign is an equation: A piece of cloth divided into thirds of red, white, and blue is the flag that stands for (i.e., "equals") the French nation. "A sign," Jung (1961) tells us, "is always less than the thing it points to, and a symbol is always more than we understand at first sight" (p. 212). He goes on to say that we never really "invent" our symbols. In fact, the most pregnant symbols come from a vast symbolic storehouse—the collective unconscious. What we invent are often signs, which just stand for or point to something outside themselves. But a symbol is larger and more mysterious: It tempts us to stay with it, to ponder it, because it offers the promise that, since it is inexhaustible, it will yield up more than is revealed at first sight.

Dream symbols, Jung insists, are *not* equations. Any interpretive attempt to make them equations (for example, cup always and only equals vagina) vitiates symbols by turning them into signs. I believe that this kind of reductionism may appear to give meaning and order but at the cost of richness and resonance. It also falsifies one of the great psychological truths that Freud proclaimed: the multivalence, complexity, and overdetermination we find in psychic life. I mistrust any attempt to shut off surplus meaning by saying X always and only equals Y.

One test of a living symbol is that it points to something unknown (Jung, 1955): "Symbols are the best possible formulation of an idea whose referent is not clearly known" (p. 468, n. 54). But although a symbol is too complex to yield up its meaning immediately, it reveals more of itself in time. And, unlike the psychoanalytic view of the unconscious, Jungians believe that the symbol is unclear not because it must disguise its nefarious purposes but because it is so complex and ultimately unknowable. Let me give an example:

I am thinking of a metaphor that took the form of a dream image presented to me by a an aging and discouraged male patient. He dreamed of a beached whale that was encrusted with barnacles and had several holes in its head. It was being held by a woman in a beach chair, who put her arm around the whale and comforted him. But eventually she got tired and left, and the whale had—somehow—to find his way back to the water. The immediate associations pointed to this distressed, beat-up whale as embodying the patient's sense of himself, and his fears that although I was "holding him" metaphorically I would find this too taxing. (My private association was to the white whale, Moby Dick, in Melville's great novel, of whom Captain Ahab says, "He heaps me, he tasks me.") But I knew that these first associations did not exhaust the meaning of the dream symbol. The whale image hovered in the air between us for months, and gradually, though we never exhausted it, we came to see more of what this symbol meant. We talked not only of the decrepitude of this particular whale, but of the physical power that whales have (my patient was a large and physically powerful man), their teasing mystery (a mammal that lives in the sea, bears its young live, suckles them), their potential for awe and for reminding us of our kinship with the denizens of the deep. And, I was confident, there would be more that we could never plumb.

Jung makes a very important point that is, in a way, the underpinning for this entire book. He (Jung, 1921) says

> Every psychic product, if it is the best possible expression at the moment for a fact as yet unknown or only relatively known, may be regarded as a symbol, provided that we accept the expression as standing for something that is only divined and not yet clearly conscious. (p. 475)

I want to emphasize "*may be regarded* as a symbol," because it speaks to the view that meaning is constructed depending on the *attitude* one takes toward one's experience. Jung (1921) avers that whether or not something is a symbol depends on "the *attitude* of the observing consciousness. . . . on whether it regards a given fact not merely as such but also as an expression for something unknown" (p. 475). So one person's factual statement can become symbolic for someone else. The symbolic attitude, generally, is one that asks, "What larger meaning is at work here? What else is this besides what it appears to be?" It is the capacity, to reverse Marianne Moore's dictum in her poem "Poetry," to see the "imaginary toads" in the "real gardens."

Case Example

A patient tells me she and her sons are building a pond in their yard. Suddenly, a tortoise appears from nowhere. It cannot be kept in the pond. It moves according to its own slow pace. When you try to lure it out from under a bush, it will not be budged. When you least expect it, it is there. It lumbers and is silent.

The tortoise is first and foremost a real creature, not a dream image or a hallucination. In fact, the palpability of the tortoise is what is so marvelous. But to those who are drawn by temperament and training to see the "something more," the tortoise is a natural symbol or metaphor. What it is a symbol of, my patient and I do not yet know. I do know that no matter how we work on this tortoise, its meaning will not be exhausted. Indeed, often with such pregnant material, especially when it comes in dream images, "working on the image" may even be counterproductive and rob a strongly affective experience of its color. In such instances, beyond listening to the patient's associations I do very little interpreting. For it seems to me again and again that in merely contemplating the symbol together, with proper awe, the two of us enter into the penumbra of its meaning.

In this particular instance, my patient had been for some months telling me of her active life as a hematologist, preoccupied for many of her 39 years with doing and making. Even creating the pond was one such "doing." But something mysterious and surprising had come out of it, just as she had found herself in the course of the therapy changing in ways she could not account for or program herself to repeat. It was clear to us both that we could look at the tortoise as another way of being, another principle at work in the psyche—slow, patient, obeying its own inner law, not to be forced or entreated. I did not say, nor did I even think tortoise = unconscious. This would have been a gross oversimplification. What I thought was, "This tortoise can be looked on as a mysterious gift, and its very essence is its mysteriousness, its 'otherness,' its refusal to be known."

The tortoise was a real, palpable visitant in the real world. It was not a metaphor created by either the patient or myself. Just as sometimes a cigar is only a cigar, sometimes a tortoise is only a tortoise. But for those of us who choose to help create meaning for ourselves and our patients, such tortoises will readily evoke the sense of "something more." I am awed when such pregnant symbols either from dreams or from "real life" present themselves in the therapeutic hour. A hush of mutual contemplation occurs, and something peculiar happens to time. It seems to cease to exist or to become infinitely expanded. This quality of uncanniness, of being out of time and the everyday world, of entering the realm of the numinous—these are the cues that my patient and I have jointly entered the domain of the symbolic.

DIMENSIONS OF THE SYMBOLIC ATTITUDE: AWARENESS AND FREEDOM FROM ARBITRATINESS

We have just looked at two "living symbols"—one from a dream (the old whale) and one from real life (the vagrant tortoise). In each case, the symbol appeared to present itself from outside the conscious volition of the experiencing subject. But what about images and symbols that have a greater degrees of conscious intention in their use? What about the metaphors introduced by our patients and by us? Are these symbols? Whether they are symbols or not depends partly on our attitude toward them, as I have tried to show. But it also depends on how much meaning they open up or foreclose, how arbitrary or how "natural" they are. Thus a sign seems to narrow meanings to just one, to insist on the literalness of the equation A equals B. One example is a flashing yellow semaphore. There is nothing intrinsic about the connection between this signal and the need for caution, but we have adopted a convention that gives this signal a single meaning: slow down. The form of national flags is also decided by fiat or agreement. So is the form of most words, where an arbitrary sound pattern is assigned a specific meaning. The metaphors used by patients and more artfully by poets, however, do not narrow meaning but do just the opposite. They open meaning up. The metaphors that most arrest us may be those that at first glance seem startling or even arbitrary but later turn out to have multiple referents that illuminate experience. Poets offer better case material here than patients do because they are so skillful and canny in their use of symbolic material. I am thinking of Marianne Moore's metaphor (cited in Rubinstein, 1972) of a lion having a "ferocious chrysanthemum head." In this instance, a metaphor that at first seems jarring and perhaps even arbitrary appears on further scrutiny to be witty and appropriately complex. This metaphor (lion's head = ferocious chrysanthemum; or, less radically, "lion's ferocious head = chrysanthemum) startles us. Perhaps it reflects the archetypal linguistic connection I have cited (Kugler, 1982) that marries flowers and devouring. But it is not accidental; the poet, whatever the deep source of her inspiration, presumably shaped this image, subjected it to scrutiny, and allowed it to stand.

Nor is this image arbitrary. The multiple curving strands of a lion's mane do have a perceptible relation to the shape of the intricate foliage of the flower. The wit is in juxtaposing something fierce and majestic with something delicate and decorative, enabling us to see connections we had not seen before.

But when we agree that metaphors or other symbols are nonarbitrary we must ask: "To whom?" In considering the logic of schizophrenia, Rubinstein (1972) describes a patient who said, "A saint is a cigar box." This metaphor sounds at first like a brilliant bit of dadaist poetry; but on analysis it turned out that it was based on an idiosyncratic and peculiar analogy:

> A saint is surrounded (by a halo).
> A cigar box is surrounded (by a tax band).
> Therefore, a saint is a cigar box.

This analogy is based on "predicate logic" (e.g., "I am a virgin, the Virgin Mary is a virgin, therefore I am the Virgin Mary"). But it is also arbitrary—too private to be accepted by others. It is a metaphor, to be sure, but when a vague and inessential attribute is excessively abstracted and generalized, the metaphor feels very different from one that is based on an essential if subtle shared attribute. The patient's metaphor in this case does not make you say "Oh!" or "Aha!"

In fact, in the pathologies of metaphor making we see not only arbitrariness but perhaps a true loss of deliberateness as well. The metaphor is taken in a literal way as what Melanie Klein [Segal, 1957] called a "symbolic equation." In schizophrenic thought the distinction between simile and metaphor is blurred. "My father is an armored tank," no longer becomes "a way of speaking," but a literal rendering. The pathology of metaphor on the opposite side is a different kind of literalism that says, "How can your father be an armored tank? He's not made of metal, he's not a machine. Your father is nothing but your father."

In fact, in an early, seminal paper, Searles (1962) maintains that until they begin recovery, schizophrenic patients are oblivious to the difference between the concrete and the metaphorical, "and it is this distinction that gives metaphor its richness" (p. 46). In some way, the concrete and metaphorical are fused, rather than simultaneously maintained but separated in the consciousness awareness of "as if." Searles avers, "Thus we might say that just as the schizophrenic is unable to think in consensually validated metaphor, so, too, is he unable to think in terms which are genuinely concrete, free from an animistic kind of so-called metaphorical overlay" (p. 23). This kind of failure of abstract attitude is seen in a patient's response to proverbs. In being told by Searles, "You can't have your cake and eat it too!" a male patient responded, "I don't want to eat any cake in this hospital." Searles maintains that the concrete interpretation of the metaphorical statement allowed the patient to avoid dealing with the unpleasant emotional meaning of the statement. Indeed, Searles believes that all such metaphorical impairments represented defenses against intolerable emotional contents.

The pathologies of symbol-making include on the one hand the loss of awareness of "as if," with the equals sign taken literally (the symbolic equation); and on the other side, the inability to take the "as if" attitude at all—a hyperfactual stance in which meaning is leached out of experience. We will presently see these poles reflected in difficulties in symbolic play. When the symbolic equation is taken concretely, it cannot bridge domains. When it is rejected because it does not make literal sense, again it cannot bridge domains. In either case, the linking or transcending power of symbolic connection is vitiated.

FAILURES OF THE CAPACITY
TO SYMBOLIZE

We can call these failures by different names: failures of the symbolic attitude, failure in the ability to play, or failure in the ability to imagine. Plaut (1966) has classified patients who have such difficulties in imagining into two categories:

1. The patient who lacks a central ego core, so that bits of passive imagery like dreams or fantasies exist, but they do not seem to belong to anyone. Plaut (1966) ascribes this dissociation to the failure of the maternal environment to hold the infant during periods of excitement. The analyst must do this for the adult patient and must also help find imagery "which is appropriate and can eventually . . . be expressed in words and thus linked with the conscious part of the ego" (p. 116). This experience of the past in the present—or perhaps re-experiencing the past in a different present—is necessary for the sense of one's own reality. The trust in one's own reality comes from trusting in another, from the experience that the other does not exist in disconnected pieces.

2. The patient who can form images and can identify them as his or hers but cannot trust them. The patient has been forced prematurely to grow up. In presenting the case history of one such patient, Plaut writes, "Unlike other children she had never learned to play, she had only become clever" (p. 118). In the course of the treatment, this patient developed severe oedipal fantasies about the analyst's wife, family, and other patients. But she truncated the fantasies on pragmatic grounds, asking, "What good are these fantasies? They lead nowhere." This patient's acceptance of a prematurely adult stance in her family had made her feel useful and desirable but

at the price of keeping her infantile sexual and destructive fantasies split off. The depreciation of these fantasies was her defense against their enormous and even quasi-delusional strength, allowing her to preserve the illusion that by rigidly disciplining herself and by being "sensible," she could become the omnipotent special child of her parents.

Jung (1951) talks in *Aion* about these two kinds of symbolizing difficulties as pathologies in the relation of the ego to the Self (the totality of the personality). If the ego is absorbed by the Self, reality perception is severely threatened. (This happens in a smaller way when the ego comes under the influence of an unconscious factor like an autonomous complex that seems to "possess" a person temporarily and whose power Jung attributed to its archetypal core). If the Self is absorbed by the ego, as in Plaut's second example, the resulting inflation leads to pride at one's control and the omnipotence of one's own will. In neither case is oscillating between the poles possible; the person is unable to make fantasy become imagination by being linked with the pole of reality.

If we try to imagine the childhood "play" experiences of the two kinds of relation to the symbolic, we see that in each case the other pole has collapsed (see Ogden, 1986). In order to play house, for example, the child must be able to shift between (1) being committed to (and therefore at times at one with) her creations or symbols, and (2) knowing that these symbols or percepts are constructed, are "as-if." When the reality pole collapses, the child is left only with symbolic equivalents. She believes while playing house that she is only the mother and this is actually her house. This is delusion.

At the other pole is the child who plays house and knows at every minute during her play that she is only a little girl playing house. In such constriction, the "as-if" experience does not take place. Instead of symbolizing, there is the "nothing but" of reality and the controlling ego. The "as-if" or symbolizing experience requires that fantasy and reality not be split off from each other but that two contradictory positions must be held in tension: "I am the mother" and at the same time "I am a little girl." This tension of asserted opposites reminds me of Winnicott's paradox of the transitional object: "I made it/I found it," or "Mother and I are one/Mother and I are two."

Identification with the Symbolic

In a total identification with the symbolic, the ego is absorbed into the unconscious. The most extreme forms of such identification occur in psychotic or borderline states where the ego gets lost in or swamped by unconscious contents. But such identification can exist in more encapsulated ways in better-functioning patients. I take an example from a middle-aged patient of Rosemary Gordon, one of the London group of Jungians. Gordon (1978) describes her patient as producing abundant material in her dreams and associations and in the transference revealing her unconscious identification with the Great Mother. The patient was so identified with this archetype that she acted out the Great Mother with her adolescent daughter by trying to give to her and to control her in a superhuman way. The daughter complied by becoming psychosomatically ill, bedridden, and helpless. The process of disidentifying with unconscious contents requires that the ego must be helped to disengage, to step aside and note what is happening as an "as-if" rather than being immersed in or possessed by the complex.

Gordon (1978) describes the analytic work on this complex as follows:

> Only when, as a result of analysis, a disidentification with this archetypal image had occurred, could the patient herself begin to develop, could a person emerge with an individual identity; only then could she begin to tolerate some change, some growth, some separateness, acknowledge the different needs of different persons, and become aware that children at different states of their development need a different type of mothering. Then could she also begin to relate herself to the helpless and hurt and frightened child inside her. This then broke up, at last, the matriarchal pattern that had gripped her family for three generations. (p. 112)

Identification with the Ego

Milner (1957) describes the opposite problem. Milner states that what impedes the imaginative life of many psychoanalytic patients is the failure of the child's early environment to provide the opportunity for "absentmindedness" or reverie—a state in which one does not distinguish between seer and seen. In this stage of "illusion" as infants and children, we may produce things that look like madness, but we are not necessarily displaying symptoms. Instead, we may be creating symbols that can be used through daydreaming or getting "lost" in play.

Patients who say "A thing either is or it isn't" are those for whom the literal meaning of something is the *only* meaning. It is likely that they have experienced the excessive early impingement of controlling or disturbed parents as their own disturbance. This forces them to construct boundaries rigidly and prematurely and leads to a precocious flattened "realism." Such a reductive adaptation, Milner says, often occurs when a parent is mentally ill, which forces the child to cling to the me/not-me distinction as the only protection against being fused with the disturbed parent.

Ego mastery introduced too early is associated with the belief in omnipotent control that we see in so many super-factual, rational, skeptical "nothing-but" patients. Milner herself gives what is now a classic case example of just such a patient whom she worked with as a young boy: In "Aspects of Symbolization in Comprehension of the Not-Self" (Milner, 1952), she describes the treatment of an 11-year-old boy who had suffered early losses including the absence of his father at war just at the time his brother was born, the loss of his residence during the bombing of London, and the loss of a favorite toy—a soft rabbit that had been his beloved transitional object. All these impingements as well as a very unsatisfactory early feeding schedule forced him to take a stance of fortitude and self-control: He became the little man of the family. But the strain began to show, and difficulties at school led to his being seen in treatment.

Milner (1952) notes that the child took a quasi-sadistic, hectoring tone toward her, which disappeared when he played with toys in her consulting room. In play, he had a different relationship to reality, which caused her to remember her own process in doing the free drawings she later described in *On Not Being Able to Paint* (1957). Somehow that play took place midway between dream or reverie and purposeful long-range action. It was a kind of oscillation, each new play conformation setting off new possibilities, just as in painting a mark on the canvas suggests another mark. There is a rhythm of "regression" and "progression."

In the countertransference, Milner (1952) experienced herself as the boy's possession (his lost rabbit) or as an extension of himself: "He so often treated me as totally his own to do what he liked with, as though I were dirt, his dirt, or as a tool, an extension of his own hand. . . . it certainly did seem that for a very long time he did need to have the illusion that I was part of himself" (p. 187). The child in fact seemed to oscillate between an illusion of union (we are one) and the fact of contact (we are two).

It was Milner's allowing of him to use her as an object or extension of himself that eventually helped him transform his play. This play initially consisted of setting fire to toy villages. In its later elaborations, as he gained trust in the analyst, the play took on an almost religious quality, as he would repeatedly light tiers of candles in play rituals reminiscent of ancient sacrificial rites or alchemical practices. In this dramatic and beautiful play the child became the playwright or stage manager and the analyst felt that her own imagination "caught fire" (Milner, 1952):

> It was in fact play with light and fire. He would close the shutters of the room and insist that it be lit only by candle light . . . And then he would make what he called furnaces, with a very careful choice of what ingredients should make the fire, including dried leaves from special plants in my garden; and sometimes all the ingredients had to be put in a metal cup on the electric fire and stirred continuously, all this carried out in the half darkness of candle light. And often there had to be a sacrifice, a lead soldier had to be added to the fire, and this figure was spoken of either as the victim or the sacrifice. In fact, all this type of play had a dramatic ritual quality comparable to the fertility rites described by Frazer in primitive societies. And this effect was the more striking because this boy's conscious interests were entirely conventional for his age, he was absorbed in Meccano and model railways. (p. 188)

This symbolic play had to do in its content with redeeming damaged objects. But in a formal way it had to do with the boy's withdrawing cathexis from the outer world and transcending his excessively realistic ego to make a new whole. This requires a temporary giving up of the sense of oneself as separate, of the reality ego that judges and discriminates. In this "aesthetic moment" of being merged with the object of creation or contemplation, writes Milner, we recapitulate the original illusion of fusion.

Again, harking back to the frame and the symbolic, Milner (1952) talks about the ability to allow illusion (neither to be compelled by it nor to exclude it, but to *allow* it), to feel "within the enclosed space-time of the drama or the picture or the story or the analytic hour, a transcending of that common sense perception which would see a picture as only an attempt at photography or the analyst as only a present day person" (p. 190).

Milner could have chosen to see her young patient's early attempts to control her and treat her as part of himself solely as the regressive enactment of a destructive fantasy. Instead, she chose to see it as a necessary regression that was in fact forward looking. Ecstatic moments of fusion with the mother are essential if the world is to be anything other than static, gray, or literal. If the child becomes aware of his separateness too early and too continually, the result may be on the one hand chaos, or on the other, as in this case, a premature cathexis of a meager "reality."

In seeing the restitutive and even "artistic" quality of her young patient's symbolization, Milner recognized the health-promoting possibilities of primary process in the context of a holding environment. Indeed, she notes that the turning point in the analysis came when she in effect departed from the classical Fenichel-Jones view of symbolism as defensive and regressive. When she began to know in her bones that her young patient's use of her was not only defensive regression (Milner, 1952) but an "essential recurrent phase in the development of a creative relation to the world, then the whole character of the analysis changed" and the boy became able to tolerate her as a separate object (p. 194).

Rethinking this case years later, in connection with a paper she was writing on Winnicott, Milner (1978) recalled those heightened moments in the boy's play. They were characterized, she recalled, by enormous concentration and by his preoccupation with lighted candles and fires in the dark and with the visitation of the gods. She connects this play with Winnicott's "creative apperception," which is available to all of us—not just to artists. This creative apperception colors external reality "in a new way, a way that can give a feeling of great significance and can in fact, as he [Winnicott] claims, make life worth living even in the face of much instinct deprivation" (p. 40). The connection with the symbolic in oscillation with the connection to the "real world" is what adds depth, meaning, and resonance to one's experience.

PATIENTS WHO CANNOT PLAY

At the outset of their treatment, the two patients we have been looking at exemplified opposite difficulties in relating to the symbolic. The woman who was so unconsciously attached to embodying the Great Mother could not detach from her identification with the archetypal symbol. And the little boy who had become prematurely adult could not attach to symbols. Both these difficulties represent an inability to play.

The emphasis on play in life and in analysis has been a recurring theme, sounded most loudly by Winnicott. But Jung (1931a) wrote much earlier, "The creative activity of imagination frees man from his bondage to the 'nothing but' and raises him to the status of one who plays. As Schiller says, man is completely human only when he is at play" (p. 46).

And in Winnicott's (1971) famous words, "Psychotherapy takes place in the overlap of two areas of playing, that of the patient and that of the therapist. Psychotherapy has to do with two people playing together" (p. 38). He goes on to say that if the therapist cannot play "then he is unsuitable for the work." And if the patient cannot play, the therapist must direct his or her efforts toward helping the patient play, "after which psychotherapy may begin" (p. 54).

Sometimes we can have the illusion of play that turns out to be only a forced compliance, an attempt at ingratiation on the patient's part. Patients cannot and should not be forced to play. An example (see Chapters 4 and 7) is the man I have called Howard L. His early metaphoric image of himself (a jar of jelly beans) got stalled because he saw its elaboration as merely an attempt to please me and rightly resisted that impulse. Indeed, it was the analysis of this interaction that allowed him to understand how common was this pattern of overt submission and covert defiance; as he learned to be more directly critical of me, he was freer to do what he wanted to do in the hours, and the metaphors of self he finally did produce (the flow-chart, the dome, the atoms in motion) were spontaneous and moving and were accompanied by strong affect. Such affect, especially in patients with intellectualizing defenses, heralds a true symbolic engagement—real play—and not just "playing at."

I am reminded also of the patient Plaut discussed in his paper on not being able to imagine. As I have already recounted, he describes supplying image after image to a patient seen early in his career; the therapy seemed to be going swimmingly with both participants appearing to play. But there was no analysis of the transference, which would have attempted to address and repair the patient's inability to play. The patient seemed to get better, but, says Plaut (1966), the change was only superficial, and the patient's life deteriorated dramatically after he quit. "A superstructure of interesting imagery (which was temporarily effective) had been built by the patient's and analyst's joint enthusiasm, but it lacked solid foundations" (p. 130).

In many cases when a patient cannot play, it is because he or she is operating at the level of "the basic fault," where survival of the very self is at stake and where symbolic equations abound. Then the last-ditch defenses—what Fordham (1974) calls "the defenses of the Self"—are invoked. Words are then no longer the medium of communication or play but are deadly weapons hurled by the participants against each other. Anyone who has worked intensively with borderline patients has had this experience. Play is the furthest thing from anyone's mind. What is required is survival: for the therapist lashing oneself to the mast and weathering the affect storms; for the patient, learning that his words are not lethal, that both parties do survive.

ON MAKING IT SAFE TO PLAY

How can the defended, fearful, enraged, or regressed patient be helped to play? If we accept Plaut's judgment that in order to play the patient must be able to trust the therapist, then we can reframe the question. We must ask what is it that will foster the patient's trust? Because the damage to the capacity to play often occurred at a preverbal developmental stage, it needs to be repaired at a preverbal level, that is, not simply at the level of interpretation. What we strive to supply, then, is an atmosphere or environment, a space or place in which the patient can count on our steadiness, dependability, benign lack of judgment, our relative predictability and our "thereness"—that very going-on-being, as Winnicott calls it, that may have been so disrupted in the patient's infancy. One of the most important things I or any of us do as therapists is simply to be there—at the same time and place, rarely absent except for vacations announced well in advance, enduring without retaliation or coercion or hidden agendas while witnessing what the patient is suffering or experiencing. This is what makes the situation safe and what eventually will enable patients who are too frightened or constricted or awash in the unconscious to begin to play.

Case Example

A patient I saw for several years, Claire F., was an accountant, who was enormously concrete. Food and money were pretty much all she talked about for two years, and it was impossible for her to see that any of her concerns had to do with other things like being nourished or loved. I assumed that her history (mostly lost to memory) had been one of enormous maternal deprivation and of precocious need to develop a reality-ego. Since my interpretations got almost nowhere, I gave up doing anything but indicating that I was there, available for her to use as she wanted. By the end of the second year she had become increasingly comfortable with me, could occasionally joke with me, and trusted me with some of her meager early memories.

One day she talked about having recently commissioned her sister to bring her a tourmaline (her birthstone) from a recent trip to Arizona. On her return, the sister told her that she had debated between getting a perfect but somewhat lusterless stone and one that had some imperfections but was extremely lustrous. The sister had chosen the lustrous but imperfect stone. The patient thanked her for her trouble. "But you know," she confessed to me, "I almost can't help wishing she'd got the perfect, duller one. That says a lot, doesn't it?" Something about the way she said this, the wry smile and the shrug, suggested that she knew and I would know that she was talking not just about tourmalines but about herself. She was talking about her obsession with perfectionism and the price she paid for it in "luster."

For the first time, she had felt safe enough to move out from the purely concrete to the transitional realm of the symbol that could widen her experience and give it resonance and meaning. It seemed a small thing, but I regarded it as a paler version of that "Aha!" experience that Helen Keller had when she first grasped the connection between the running water and the sign Annie Sullivan was tracing on her hand. In that thrilling moment, the world of symbols opened up and enabled Helen, that nearly feral child, to become for the first time a member of the human community. To be a participant-observer at the moment when a frightened or constricted patient feels securely enough held to take her first step into the realm of symbolic play—this is being a midwife to the birth of the capacity for meaning. But in addition to a safe atmosphere or holding environment, safety has to do with the therapist's own symbolic stance, the therapist's realization that everything that takes place in the room can be read in more than one way: as conscious interpersonal exchange, as derivatives of unconscious content, as exemplifying the patient's inner object world, and as reflecting as well a real relationship. In a safe environment, the patient can be led to see how he or she is using the therapist in a symbolic way, transferring past experiences, attitudes, and projections. Once this is established, it serves as a master metaphor for both destructive and creative illusion—for the compelled repetitions and the attempts to step outside them and discover the therapist as a "new object."

Being captured by a complex is a very different experience from being just a little outside it and being able to register that fact by telling oneself, "I am possessed or caught up in this situation. This is a symbolic replay of a terribly painful earlier experience." Such a statement does not deny or dismiss the experience as simply irrational and therefore unacceptable, nor does it keep one immersed in the destructive element. It allows both for the intense, often excruciating re-experiences of loss or rage *and* nearly simultaneously for inaugurating the ability to question the meaning or affective charge that is attached to those feelings.

This to-ing and fro-ing is what the depth therapist or analyst does. It is what I do when I am working at my best: not supplying ingenious images or brilliant formulations, but groping, waiting, and oscillating. I am moving back and forth between focus and reverie, separateness and fusion, experience and comment, oscillating between here and now and there and then. This kind of oscillation attempts to mediate between conscious and unconscious, taking both poles with full seriousness and looking for the vantage point that enables us to be both inside the experience, temporarily identified with the patient, and just a little to one side. In an implicit way, I offer this stance to my patients as a model for functioning: to help them respect their own experience as well as question it, to respect their unconscious impulses as well as their conscious strivings, and to alternate between doing and being.

The master metaphor of my work draws on music. It is not so much spatial as temporal, not so much cognitive as affective. It is as concerned with form as with content. Or rather it is concerned with the form of content. How the story is told is as important as what is told. How a dream is presented is as important as what is presented: Is it a gift? A supplication? A challenge? Is it thrown away as garbage? Is it a narcissistic delight—the child proudly presenting his feces to his mother—"Look what I made?" Is it a gauntlet thrown down ("See what you can make of this crazy thing")? Is it a deluge (five dreams in an hour and both of us gasping for breath)?

When you attend to the how of a presentation, the "music" becomes paramount. I can only talk about this metaphorically because there is no literal "music" in the room, but the quality of music, and its connection with feeling is notable by its absence or presence. One therapist who clearly understands about such music is Robert Hobson, whose interaction with his patient Freda around the metaphor of "the empty heart" I described in Chapter 6. Hobson (1986) writes of the therapist's music of the "Mmm" or the "Ah":

> I remember other occasions in therapy, when a long drawn-out "Ah" has been heard as something like a melody, or even a fugue with a harmonizing of different verbal, tonal, and non-verbal "voices." In conversation we use many channels of communications hoping for a resolution of discords. A psychotherapist needs assiduous practice in using the wide-ranging language of "Mm." It can be a highly imaginative creation. (p. 23)

THE SYMBOLIC ATTITUDE AND THE
AESTHETIC ATTITUDE

Literally, the aesthetic has to do with appreciating or responding to the beautiful in art or nature, derived from *aiesthetes*, one who perceives. Perhaps the classical Freudian uneasiness about art derives in part from Freud's own acknowledgment that he felt unable to register "aesthetic emotion." He was enormously interested in the arts, but primarily as texts to provide illustrations or to require explication. His cherished artifacts and his wide reading needed to eventuate in a message. Freud also said, according to Susan Deri (1978), that he took almost no pleasure in music. This is not surprising since very little in music illustrates or points to anything. The form or sensuous surface—the *made* aspects of the arts were not engaging to Freud: They had to point to—preferably to point down to—something hidden. Thus, Deri avers, Freud could not appreciate the creative nature of the manifest dream.

Winnicott, on the other hand, felt that art was essential to a full life. His wife Clare Winnicott (1978) notes in a reminiscence that not only did he play the piano briefly between sessions and at the end of the day but that

> Donald's knowledge and appreciation of music was a joy to both of us . . . He always had a special feeling for the music of Bach but at the end of his life it was the late Beethoven string quartets that absorbed and fascinated him. It seems as if the refinement and abstraction in the musical idiom of these works helped him to gather in and realise in himself the rich harvest of a lifetime. (p. 30)

This affinity for the arts—especially music—allowed him to attend to transitional phenomena not as mere "sublimations" but as that sphere of life which has its own vital energy—the sphere of art, culture, and religion. It was this conviction that caused him to write so fully about transitional phenomena and play, the space of creating as well as finding.

Winnicott (1971) has written that a quotation from Tagore, "On the seashore of endless worlds children play," haunted him for years before he used it as the epigraph of his essay on "The Location of

Cultural Experience." That is not surprising, for the phrase embodies much of what Winnicott stands for: "Endless worlds" suggests the opening out of creative possibility; "children play" became the focus of his work. And "the seashore" is a perfect metaphor for liminal or transitional space: Is it land or is it sea? Is it here or is it there? The visible shoreline shifts as the tides move in and out. It is that mysterious transitional space which is metaphorically the meeting of two elements: land and sea, outer world and inner world, conscious and unconscious.

But beyond the content, the Tagore quotation has a mysterious resonance that cannot be exhausted by simply glossing the words. Much of this has to do with the formal inversion of the phrase. The line would *say* the same thing if it read "Children play on the seashore of endless worlds." But the *music* would be gone, and instead we would have something like an empirical observation. The delaying of the subject and verb to the end of the line ("On the seashore of endless worlds, children play) recasts it from a statement of fact to a feeling-toned music. And that feeling-toned music is experienced in the therapeutic exchange as resonance.

A MUSICAL METAPHOR OF THE THERAPEUTIC ENCOUNTER: RESONANCE AND ATTUNEMENT

Our key metaphors are really our signatures. Because music has always been my main nonhuman source of joy and consolation, it becomes my hallmark of affective experience. Langer (1948) described music as the language of the emotions. It makes sense that the metaphor of the therapeutic process that I find most congenial—especially when the process is working well—comes from a nonmaterial art like music rather than from the realm of material objects be they archeological, geological, geographical; be they frames, vessels, or containers. All of these are suggestive and useful, but they describe a surround or an atmosphere rather than the very lively activity that occurs in that surround. I need a metaphor that is more active and more interactive, that emphasizes mutuality and that suggests movement in time. The metaphors I often experience in my work are musical metaphors: The two participants are in relationship as dancers or instrumentalists are.

Oliver Sacks (1984) quotes the German philosopher Novalis as saying, "Every disease is a musical problem, every cure a musical solution" (p. 137). Something about our patients has become unstrung and discordant, and they need a resonant responder to restore something that got jammed along the way—a "rhythm of safety" (the beautiful phrase comes from Frances Tustin, 1987).

I once marveled to an analyst of mine, trying to account for the intense and mysterious feelings generated in the room, "It's amazing. We're only two people talking." And he said, "Yes, but that leaves out the resonance." It occurred to me then that to describe a therapeutic encounter as "two people talking," says as little about the music of the exchange as saying a string quartet is four people using horsehair to scrape across catgut. All reductionism, all nothing-but formulations leave out the resonance.

What is this resonance? The resonance is the affect and the communication from unconscious to unconscious. It is everything that cannot be revealed in a bare transcript: It is the tone of voice, the facial expressions and body language, the web of connotation that a particular word touches off in patient and therapist, who jointly develop a common idiom. This resonance creates the ripples that radiate out from what the patient reveals. It is what allows us to see the imaginary toads in the real gardens. When a patient talks about the tortoise that mysteriously appeared near her pond, we both know it was a real tortoise and a real pond. And yet as we talk, we see how much the turtle is not only a turtle but represents something else whose meaning we can only guess at. The mutual recognition of the "something more" that we cannot fully know feels resonant because it opens up layers of latent meaning.

This resonance is what causes us to dream about patients and them to dream about us. It is what permits at times a "harmonious interpenetrating mixup" (in Balint's phrase) that makes it hard to tell who did what and to whom. If one thinks of the therapist as "attuned," one sees parallels to the good-enough mother's attunement to the infant which requires not only "reverie" and "maternal preoccupation" but exquisite sensitivity to nonverbal cues: body movements, facial expressions, precise nuances of the sort that distinguishes a cry of hunger from a cry of pain or irritation or anger. All these cues—including the registration of mismatch between the words and the music (a patient tells you how anxious she is about her floundering law practice while she is grinning)—are our stock in trade. And any therapeutic metaphor that casts the encounter in purely verbal terms leaves out the other signals of affect that are at least as important. It is not a choice between the cognitive and the affective; it is a combination. Not either/or, but both/and.

For me, an inability to register these cues or a sense that only one person is dancing while I am merely watching from the sidelines suggests that something has gone awry either in my empathic capacities at that moment or in the patient's capacity for relatedness. When therapy is mutually engaging, it often feels like a dance: sometimes an erotic tango, sometimes a wild tarantella, sometimes a slow saraband or pavane, sometimes an aikido-like standoff. At times, the therapist leads unobtrusively. At other times, the patient may lead but the therapist is a partner. Sometimes it is hard to say just who is leading. Perhaps it is correct to say that the unconscious is leading, evoking mutually similar associations.

One index that things are moving well is that my next silent association or fantasy anticipates—without any willed effort on my part—what the patient's next association will be. A woman describes writing an angry letter to a complete stranger met only at a charity ball. My patient feels this woman is a phony and a superstar. I think, "Sister stuff in here . . . and something about these qualities in herself." Her next association is to her sister's upstaging of her. And a little later in the hour she talks about her sensitivity to impostors and her own fear that *she* is a phony. Other moments are more like merger—seeing oneself in the patient, the patient in oneself; these moments, like music, exist in time but permit a sense of timelessness in a heightened present.

Are these experiences of words or of music? They are both, of course. There is no reason to deprive oneself of words while attending to the music. In fact, it is the interaction or congruence that is all-important. If Schubert had set the melody of his song, "Death and the Maiden," to the words of "Twinkle, Twinkle Little Star," the result would have been a gross misalliance. Song, in fact, may be a good analogy for the therapeutic process because it depends for its effect on the union of words and music. The texts of songs, which draw on highly charged verse, are themselves a verbal music. One would not set a legal document or an environmental impact statement to music. And this fact may give us a cue—when we are getting from our patients some version of a legal document or environmental impact statement, or the news of the week in review, we ask, "Where is the music? Where is the passion behind the prose?"

Case Example: From Mechanism to Music

I would like to conclude with a literal musical example from the case of a man I'll call Roger F., who was almost completely "unmusicked." Indeed, his affect was so uniformly and hollowly cheerful and his style so pedantic that I came to think of him as "The Mechanical Man."

I saw Roger, a 34-year-old mechanical engineer, in a short-term focused way that is atypical of my usual therapeutic mode; this way of working was all he could accept at the time. He wanted help with a specific crisis: He was about to be fired from his job. Roger had read my book on psychological change and risk-taking (Siegelman, 1983) and come to a workshop I was giving on the subject. In the course of filling out a questionnaire I had devised on risk-taking styles, he unknowingly established the construct validity of my brief test. He scored all ten items in the direction of the "anxious risk-taker" (basically an extremely obsessional style). As I later learned from his history, he was even more constricted and ruminative than the exaggerated prototype I had constructed.

In the course of his 8-months therapy, he would characteristically utter mechanical interjections like "Not to worry," or "Sorry about that." I would find myself at times wondering, "How does one relate to a robot?" I suppose the answer was that almost from the start I felt the extraordinary woundedness that all his armor was designed to protect. Sharing this knowledge with him was very difficult since, despite his brilliance and the inventiveness of his science-fiction fantasies, he could not process interpretations of affect. The resonance came in for me when I could hear the unconscious reverberations of some of his statements: He had joined a medieval jousting society but had to quit, he told me, "because my armor is too thin."

The unacknowledged metaphor behind this statement I experienced as extremely poignant. I saw this man's obsessional defenses as covering a very vulnerable schizoid orientation. My inner experience was much like what Searles (1962) describes in dealing with "the stressful experience of sensing poignant metaphorical meanings in the patient's remarks, messages which the patient is as yet unaware of conveying, messages having an affective impact with which the therapist must cope, therefore, in a state of felt aloneness" (p. 41). He maintains that this is an experiencing in the countertransference of the kind of aloneness the patient as a child must have felt when his early attempts at grasping metaphorical meanings of things were met by the parents' unconscious denial of these kinds of meanings. I had to do what Searles says one must do in such situations—putting the metaphor on hold while talking with the patient in the only terms presently available to him or her—that is, literal terms.

Since attempts to reach his underlying feelings produced nothing but a polite acknowledgment, I was impelled to use his language—the language of cognition—to develop and share with him some ideas about his perfectionism and how it was standing in his way. This perfectionism had been so crippling that it had led to endless procrastinating, to quitting a technical school after he got one B+ (instead of his invariable A's), quitting organizations if he goofed up even once by being late, and so on. Together, we worked on his developing a range rather than a point of acceptability, and he was enormously pleased that he could come to tolerate performance that was 95 to 100 percent correct, not just 100 percent. He gradually resolved the job problem.

In the meantime, the sessions often had a bizarre quality. During one of them, preparatory to writing a paper on the subject, he gave me a 50-minute lecture on arms control. He did not think this at all odd and told me he "liked having someone to try his ideas out on." This very partial, focused therapy seemed to help Roger enormously in the specific arena for which he had sought help. After eight months, he had recouped at work and was being considered for a promotion. The therapy did not restructure his psyche, but both of us were satisfied with this very real change. He acknowledged that he had more work to do about "relating to people," but would do that, he said, another time.

I increasingly respected his need for the defenses he had evolved in being a child prodigy in a family of cold, mechanical parents. I became fond of him and could empathize with the poignancy of keeping going in a world that was safe only to the extent that it was a human and emotional Sahara. We both knew that he had a long way to go in countering the aversiveness with which he experienced other people; perhaps one small dent had been made by virtue of his beginning ability to trust me.

Shortly before his last session, Roger talked to me about a folk-singing group he had joined as part of his effort to "do more things with people." He told me about the songs people sang or made up and then said, suddenly, "I'd like to sing you one." It was probably because his termination date was imminent that he could allow himself to do something so uncharacteristic and self-exposing.

Roger cleared his throat. Then he closed his eyes, and a strange thing happened: His face was suddenly suffused with light. In a high, pure tenor voice, he sang me a song about human loneliness. In singing the song, he was simultaneously confessing, connecting, and giving me a gift. I heard the metaphor as well as the song. Or rather, I heard the metaphor *in* the song, and I know he could see how deeply I was moved by this singular display of his inner music.

I believe that an essential part of what we do as therapists is to help patients recover their own inner music. The therapist's capacity to modulate from sustained attention to reverie, from cognitive interpretations to empathic identification is itself a kind of music. One hopes that our unstrung patients will eventually be able to mirror this process of flexible oscillation in their own psychic life and in this way will learn to sing the songs that are uniquely theirs.

References

Adler, G. (1951). Notes regarding the dynamics of the Self. *British Journal of Medical Psychology*, *24*, 97–106.

Aleksandrowicz, D. R. (1962). The meaning of metaphor. *Bulletin of the Menninger Clinic*, *26*, 92–101.

Arlow, J. A. (1969a). Fantasy, memory, and reality testing. *Psychoanalytic Quarterly*, *38*, 28–51.

Arlow, J. A. (1969b). Unconscious fantasy and disturbances of conscious experience. *Psychoanalytic Quarterly*, *38*, 1–27.

Arlow, J. A. (1979). Metaphor and the psychoanalytic situation. *Psychoanalytic Quarterly*, *48*, 363–385.

Auden, W. H. (1976). *Collected poems* (Ed. E. Mendelson). New York: Random House.

Balint, M. (1968). *The basic fault: Therapeutic aspects of regression*. London: Tavistock.

Barlow, J. M., Pollio, H. R., & Fine, H. J. (1977). Insight and figurative language in psychotherapy. *Psychotherapy: Theory, Research, and Practice*, *14*, 212–222.

Beck, A. T. (1967). *Depression: Causes and treatment*. Philadelphia: University of Pennsylvania Press.

Bruner, J. (1986). Thought and emotion: Can Humpty Dumpty be put together again? In D. Bearison & H. Zimiles (Eds.), *Thought and emotion* (pp. 11–20). Hillsdale, NJ: Erlbaum.

Cain, A. C., & Maupin, B. M. (1961). Interpretation within the metaphor. *Bulletin of the Menninger Clinic*, *25*, 307–311.

Carotenuto, A. (1982). *A secret symmetry: Sabina Spielrein between Jung and Freud*. New York: Pantheon.

Carroll, Lewis. (1946). *Through the looking glass, and what Alice found there*. New York: Random House.

Caruth, E., & Ekstein, R. (1966). Interpretation within the metaphor. *Journal of the American Academy of Psychiatry*, *5*, 35–45.

Carveth, D. (1984). The analyst's metaphors: A deconstructionist perspective. *Psychoanalysis and Contemporary Thought*, *7*, 491–560.

Dennison, G. (1985). *Luisa Domic*. New York: Harper & Row.

Deri, S. (1978). Transitional phenomena: Vicissitudes of symbolization and creativity. In S. A. Grolnick & L. Barkin, (Eds.), *Between reality and fantasy: Transitional objects and phenomena* (pp. 43–60). New York: Jason Aronson.

Doolitle, H. ["H.D."] (1984). *Tribute to Freud*. New York: New Directions.

Ekstein, R., & Wallerstein, J. (1956). Observations on the psychotherapy of borderline and psychotic children. *Psychoanalytic Study of the Child, 11*, 303–311.

Eliot, T. S. (1929). Dante. In *Selected essays, 1917–1932*. New York: Harcourt Brace, 1933.

Eliot, T. S. (1963). *Collected poems, 1909–1962*. New York: Harcourt Brace.

Field, J. (pseudonym of Marion Milner) (1936). *A life of one's own*. Los Angeles: J. P. Tarcher, 1981.

Field, J. (pseudonym of Marion Milner) (1937). *An experiment in leisure*. Los Angeles: J. P. Tarcher, 1987.

Fisher, S. (1970). *Body experience in fantasy and behavior*. New York: Appleton-Century-Crofts.

Fisher, S., & Cleveland, S. E. (1968). *Body image and personality*. (2nd ed., rev.). New York: Dover.

Fordham, M. (1974). Defences of the self. *Journal of Analytical Psychology, 19*, 192–199.

Forrest, D. V. (1973). On one's own onymy. *Psychiatry, 36*, 266–290.

Forster, E. M. (1921). *Howard's end*. New York: Vintage.

Freud, S. (1900). The interpretation of dreams. *Standard Edition, 5*. London: Hogarth Press, 1953.

Freud, S. (1909). Notes upon a case of obsessional neurosis. *Standard Edition, 10*, pp. 153–318. London: Hogarth Press, 1955.

Freud, S. (1911). Formulations regarding the two principles in mental functioning. In *Collected papers* (Vol. 4). New York: Basic Books, 1959.

Freud, S. (1919). Lines of advance in psychoanalytic therapy. *Standard Edition, 17*. London: Hogarth Press, 1955.

Freud, S. (1923). *The ego and the id*. New York: W. W. Norton, 1962.

Freud, S. (1929). Civilization and its discontents. *Standard Edition, 21*, pp. 64–145. London: Hogarth Press, 1961.

Freud, S. (1933). New introductory lectures on psycho-analysis. *Standard Edition, 22*. London: Hogarth Press, 1964.

Freud, S. (1937). Analysis terminable and interminable. *Standard Edition, 23*, pp. 216–253. London: Hogarth Press, 1959.

Gardner, H., with Winner, E. (1982). The child as father to the metaphor. In H. Gardner, Art, mind and brain: A cognitive approach to creativity. New York: Basic Books.

Goodheart, W. B. (1980). Theory of analytic interaction. San Francisco Jung Institute Library Journal, 1(4), 2–39.

Goodheart, W. B. (1984). C. G. Jung's first 'patient': On the seminal emergence of Jung's thought. Journal of Analytical Psychology, 29 (1), 1–34.

Gordon, R. (1978). Dying and creating: A search for meaning. Library of Analytical Psychology, Vol. 4. London: Society of Analytical Psychology.

Hobson, R. F. (1986). Forms of feeling: The heart of psychotherapy. London: Tavistock.

Johnson, M. (1987). The body in the mind: The bodily basis of meaning, imagination, and reason. Chicago: University of Chicago Press.

Jones, E. (1916). The theory of symbolism. In Papers on psychoanalysis. London: Bailliere, Tindall, & Cox, 1950.

Jung, C. G. (1916). The transcendent function. In H. Read, M. Fordham, G. Adler, & W. McGuire, (Eds.), The Collected Works of C. G. Jung, 8, Bollingen Series 20, 67–92. Princeton: Princeton University Press, 1960.

Jung, C. G. (1921). Psychological types. Collected Works, 6. Princeton: Princeton University Press, 1971.

Jung, C. G. (1929). Introduction to The Secret of The Golden Flower. Collected Works, 12, 1–56. Princeton: Princeton University Press, 1967.

Jung, C. G. (1931a). The aims of psychotherapy. Collected Works, 16, 36–52. Princeton: Princeton University Press.

Jung, C. G. (1931b). On the relation of analytical psychology to poetry. Collected Works, 15, 63-83. Princeton: Princeton University Press, 1966.

Jung, C. G. (1935). The Tavistock lectures. Collected Works, 18, 1-182. Princeton: Princeton University Press, 1980.

Jung, C. G. (1944). Psychology and Alchemy (2nd ed.). Collected Works, 12. Princeton: Princeton University Press, 1968.

Jung, C. G. (1946). The psychology of the transference. Collected Works, 16, 163-323. Princeton: Princeton University Press, 1966.

Jung, C. G. (1951) Aion: Researches into the phenomenology of the self. Collected Works, 9(2). Princeton: Princeton University Press, 1959.

Jung, C. G. (1952) Symbols of Transformation (2nd ed.). Collected Works, 5. Princeton: Princeton University Press, 1956.

Jung, C. G. (1955). Mysterium coniuncitionis. *Collected Works, 14,* Princeton: Princeton University Press.

Jung, C. G. (1961) Symbols and the interpretation of dreams. *Collected Works, 18,* 185–264. Princeton: Princeton University Press, 1980.

Jung, C. G., & Riklin, F. (1906). The associations of normal subjects. In Jung, *Collected Works, 2,* 3–195. Princeton: Princeton University Press, 1973.

Kohut, H. (1984). *How does analysis cure?* A. Goldberg (Ed.) with P. E. Stepansky. Chicago: University of Chicago Press.

Kris, E. (1952). On preconscious mental processes. In *Psychoanalytic explorations in art* (pp. 303–318). New York: International Universities Press.

Kugler, P. (1982). *The alchemy of discourse: An archetypal approach to language.* Lewisburg, PA: Bucknell University Press.

Lacan, J. (1977). *Écrits.* New York: W. W. Norton.

Lakoff, G. (1987). *Women, fire and dangerous things: What categories reveal about the mind.* Chicago: University of Chicago Press.

Lakoff, G., & Johnson, M. (1980). *Metaphors we live by.* Chicago: University of Chicago Press.

Lakoff, G., & Turner, M. (1989). *More than cool reason: A field guide to poetic metaphor.* Chicago: University of Chicago Press.

Langer, S. K. (1948). *Philosophy in a new key: A study of the symbolism of reason, rite, and art.* New York: Mentor.

Langs, R. (1978). *The listening process.* New York: Jason Aronson.

Langs, R. (1979). *The therapeutic environment.* New York: Jason Aronson.

Levenson, E. (1983). *The ambiguity of change: An inquiry into the nature of psychoanalytic reality.* New York: Basic Books.

Levin, F. M. (1980). Metaphor, affect, and arousal: How interpretations might work. *Annual of Psychoanalysis, 8,* 231–245.

Loewald, H. W. (1960). Therapeutic action of psycho-analysis. *International Journal of Psychoanalysis, 41,* 16–33.

Loewald, H. W. (1988). *Sublimation: Inquiries into theoretical psychoanalysis.* New Haven: Yale University Press.

Mahony, P. (1982). *Freud as a writer.* New York: International Universities Press.

Mahler, M. S., Pine, F., & Bergman, A. (1975). *The psychological birth of the human infant: Symbiosis and individuation.* New York: Basic Books.

Milner, M.: see Field, J., pseudonym.

Milner, M. (1952) Aspects of symbolism in comprehension of the not-self. *International Journal of Psychoanalysis, 33,* 181–195.

Milner, M. (1957). *On not being able to paint.* New York: International Universities Press, 1973.

Milner, M. (1969). *The hands of the living god.* New York: International Universities Press.

Milner, M. (1978). D. W. Winnicott and the two-way journey. In S. A. Grolnick & L. Barkin (Eds.), *Between reality and fantasy: Transitional objects and phenomena* (pp. 35–42). New York: Jason Aronson.

Milner, M. (1987). *The suppressed madness of sane men: Forty years of exploring psychoanalysis.* London: Methuen.

Nash, H. (1962). Freud and metaphor. *Archives of General Psychiatry, 7,* 25–29.

Nemerov, H. (1985). On metaphor. *New and selected essays.* Carbondale, IL: Southern Illinois University Press.

Ogden, T. H. (1986). *The matrix of the mind: Object relations and the psychoanalytic dialogue.* Northvale, NJ: Jason Aronson.

Ogden, T. H. (1989). *The primitive edge of experience.* Northvale, NJ: Jason Aronson

Ozick, C. (1986, May). On the moral necessity of metaphor. *Harper's,* 62–68.

Parker, B. (1962). *My language is me: Psychotherapy with a disturbed adolescent.* New York: Basic Books.

Pederson-Krag, G. (1956). The use of metaphor in analytical thinking. *Psychoanalytic Quarterly, 25,* 66–71.

Piaget, J. (1951). *Play, dreams, and imitation in childhood.* New York: Norton, 1962.

Piaget, J. (1954). *The construction of reality in the child.* New York: Basic Books.

Piaget, J. (1955). *The language and thought of the child.* New York: Meridian Books.

Plaut, A. (1966). Reflections about not being able to imagine. *Journal of Analytical Psychology, 11,* 113–133.

Reider, N. (1972). Metaphor as interpretation. *International Journal of Psychoanalysis, 53,* 463–469.

Rubinstein, B. B. (1972). On metaphor and related phenomena. In R. R. Holt & E. Peterfreund (Eds.), *Psychoanalysis and Contemporary Science* (pp. 70–108). New York: Macmillan.

Rycroft, C. (1979). *The innocence of dreams: A new approach to the study of dreams.* New York: Pantheon Books.

Sacks, O. (1984). *A leg to stand on.* New York: Summit Books.

Samuels, A. (1985). *Jung and the post-Jungians.* London: Routledge, Kegan, Paul.

Samuels, A. (1989). *The plural psyche: Personality, morality and the Father.* New York: Routledge, Chapman and Hall, Inc.

Schafer, R. (1976). *A new language for psychoanalysis.* New Haven: Yale University Press.

Schafer, R. (1983). *The analytic attitude.* New York: Basic Books.

Searles, H. F. (1962). The differentiation between concrete and metaphorical thinking in recovering schizophrenic patients. *Journal of the American Psychoanalytic Association, 10,* 22–49.

Santostefano, S. (1988). Process and change in child therapy and development: The concept of metaphor. In D. C. Morrison (Ed.), *Organizing early experience: Imagination and cognition in childhood* (pp. 139–172). Amityville, NY: Baywood.

Segal, H. (1957). Notes on symbol formation. *International Journal of Psychoanalysis, 38,* 391–397.

Shengold, L. (1981). Insight as metaphor. *Psychoanalytic Study of the Child, 36,* 289–306.

Siegelman, E. Y. (1983). *Personal risk.* New York: Harper & Row.

Siegelman, E. Y. (1987). The tower as artifact and symbol in Jung and Yeats. *Psychological Perspectives, 18,* 52–69.

Siegelman, E. Y. (1989). To-ing and fro-ing among the object relations theorists. [Review of Thomas Ogden's *The matrix of the mind*]. *San Francisco Jung Institute Library Journal, 9*(3), 7–20.

Spence, D. (1982). *Narrative truth and historical truth: Meaning and interpretation in psychoanalysis.* New York: Norton.

Spence, D. (1987). *The Freudian metaphor: Toward paradigm change in psychoanalysis.* New York: W. W. Norton.

Trilling, L. (1940). Freud and literature. In P. Meisel (Ed.), *Freud: A collection of critical essays* (pp. 95–111). Englewood Cliffs, NJ: Prentice Hall.

Tustin, F. (1987). "The rhythm of safety." *Autistic barriers in neurotic patients* (pp. 268–285). New Haven: Yale University Press.

Victor, G. (1977). *"Interpretations couched in mystical imagery."* Unpublished manuscript.

Voth, H. M. (1970). The analysis of metaphor. *Journal of The American Psychoanalytic Association, 18,* 599–621.

Weiss, J., Sampson, H., & the Mt. Zion Psychotherapy Research Group. (1986). *The psychoanalytic process: Theory, clinical observations, and empirical research.* New York: Guilford Press.

Winnicott, C. (1978). D.W.W.: A reflection. In S. A. Grolnick & L. Barkin (Eds.), *Between reality and fantasy: Transitional objects and phenomena* (pp. 15–34). New York: Jason Aronson.

Winnicott, D. W. (1958). *Collected papers: Through paediatrics to psychoanalysis.* London: Tavistock.

Winnicott, D. W. (1960). Parent–infant relationship. *The maturational processes and the facilitating environment.* New York: International Universities Press.

Winnicott, D. W. (1971). *Playing and reality.* London: Tavistock.

Winnicott, D. W. (1987). *Holding and interpretation: Fragment of an analysis.* (F. Jordan, Editor). New York: Grove.

Wright, K. J. T. (1976). Metaphor and symptom: A study of integration and its failure. *International Review of Psychoanalysis, 3,* 97–109.

Index